WE 242 BLA

D0587035

the**facts**

Osteoporosis

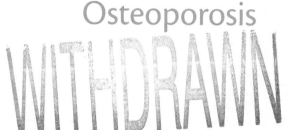

Shrewsbury Health Library

SHR03579

➲ also available in the**facts** series

Eating disorders: the**facts**
SIXTH EDITION
Abraham

Epilepsy: the**facts**
THIRD EDITION
Appleton and Marson

Osteoarthritis: the**facts**
Arden, Arden, and Hunter

Asthma: the**facts**
Arshad and Babu

Sexually transmitted infections: the**facts**
SECOND EDITION
Barlow

Autism and Asperger syndrome: the**facts**
Baron-Cohen

Epilepsy in women: the**facts**
Betts and Clarke

Living with a long-term illness: the**facts**
Campling and Sharpe

Chronic fatigue syndrome: the**facts**
SECOND EDITION
Campling and Sharpe

Head injury: the**facts**
Daisley, Tams, and Kischka

Falls: the**facts**
Darowski

Infertility: the**facts**
Davies, Overton, and Webber

Prenatal tests: the**facts**
De Crespigny and Chervenak

Obsessive-compulsive disorder: the**facts**
THIRD EDITION
de Silva

Polycystic ovary syndrome: the**facts**
Elsheikh and Murphy

Muscular dystrophy: the**facts**
THIRD EDITION
Emery

Psoriatic arthritis: the**facts**
Gladman and Chandran

The pill and other forms of hormonal
contraception: the**facts**
SIXTH EDITION
Guillebaud

Lupus: the**facts**
SECOND EDITION
Isenberg and Manzi

Ankylosing spondylitis: the**facts**
Khan

Borderline personality disorder: the**facts**
Krawitz and Jackson

Inflammatory bowel disease: the**facts**
Langmead and Irving

Stroke: the**facts**
Lindley

Diabetes: the**facts**
Matthews *et al.*

Essential tremor: the**facts**
Plumb and Bain

Huntington's disease: the**facts**
SECOND EDITION
Quarrell

Panic disorder: the**facts**
SECOND EDITION
Rachman

Tourette syndrome: the**facts**
SECOND EDITION
Robertson and Cavanna

ADHD: the**facts**
Selikowitz

Down syndrome: the**facts**
THIRD EDITION
Selikowitz

Insomnia and other adult sleep problems:
the**facts**
Stores

Sleep problems in children and adolescents:
the**facts**
Stores

Motor neuron disease: the**facts**
Talbot and Marsden

Cystic fibrosis: the**facts**
FOURTH EDITION
Thomson and Harris

Thyroid disease: the**facts**
FOURTH EDITION
Vanderpump and Tunbridge

Depression: the**facts**
Wasserman

Cosmetic surgery: the**facts**
Waterhouse

the**facts**

Osteoporosis

ALISON J. BLACK

Associate Specialist
Department of Rheumatology,
Grampian Osteoporosis Service,
Woolmanhill Hospital,
Aberdeen, UK.

RENA SANDISON

Osteoporosis Specialist Nurse
Department of Rheumatology,
Grampian Osteoporosis Service,
Woolmanhill Hospital,
Aberdeen, UK.

DAVID M. REID

Professor of Rheumatology
Division of Applied Medicine,
University of Aberdeen, UK.

OXFORD
UNIVERSITY PRESS

OXFORD
UNIVERSITY PRESS

Great Clarendon Street, Oxford OX2 6DP

Oxford University Press is a department of the University of Oxford.
It furthers the University's objective of excellence in research, scholarship,
and education by publishing worldwide in

Oxford New York

Auckland Cape Town Dar es Salaam Hong Kong Karachi
Kuala Lumpur Madrid Melbourne Mexico City Nairobi
New Delhi Shanghai Taipei Toronto

With offices in

Argentina Austria Brazil Chile Czech Republic France Greece
Guatemala Hungary Italy Japan Poland Portugal Singapore
South Korea Switzerland Thailand Turkey Ukraine Vietnam

Oxford is a registered trade mark of Oxford University Press
in the UK and in certain other countries

Published in the United States
by Oxford University Press Inc., New York

© Oxford University Press 2009

The moral rights of the authors have been asserted
Database right Oxford University Press (maker)

First published 2009

All rights reserved. No part of this publication may be reproduced,
stored in a retrieval system, or transmitted, in any form or by any means,
without the prior permission in writing of Oxford University Press,
or as expressly permitted by law, or under terms agreed with the appropriate
reprographics rights organization. Enquiries concerning reproduction
outside the scope of the above should be sent to the Rights Department,
Oxford University Press, at the address above

You must not circulate this book in any other binding or cover
and you must impose this same condition on any acquirer

British Library Cataloguing in Publication Data

Data available

Library of Congress Cataloging in Publication Data

Data available

ISBN 978-0-19-921589-8

10 9 8 7 6 5 4 3 2 1

Typeset in Plantin
by Cepha Imaging Pvt. Ltd., Bangalore, India
Printed in China through
Asia Pacific Offset

Whilst every effort has been made to ensure that the contents of this book are as complete, accurate,
and up-to-date as possible at the date of writing, Oxford University Press is not able to give any
guarantee or assurance that such is the case. Readers are urged to take appropriately qualified
medical advice in all cases. The information in this book is intended to be useful to the general
reader, but should not be used as a means of self-diagnosis or for the prescription of medication.

Preface

Osteoporosis has been termed the 'silent epidemic' of the twenty-first century. It is a condition characterized by thin bones with a subsequent increased risk of painful and disabling fractures. It is 'silent' because thin bones themselves do not cause pain and 'epidemic' because it is estimated that 1 in 2 women and 1 in 5 men are likely to suffer a fracture due to osteoporosis. The personal costs to the sufferer are clearly a concern, but so too is the economic burden of osteoporosis.

This book is intended for patients, their relatives, and carers but may also be of value to the non-specialist.

Alison Black
Rena Sandison
David Reid
Aberdeen May 2008

Contents

1

What is osteoporosis?

> ## ➡ Key points
>
> - Osteoporosis 'thin bone' results in an increased risk of fracture.
>
> - Osteoporotic fractures occur in 1 in 2 women and 1 in 5 men over the age of 50 years.
>
> - The classic sites for osteoporotic fractures are the wrist, spine and hip.
>
> - The skeleton is a metabolically active organ.
>
> - Many factors influence bone, which changes throughout life.

Osteoporosis

In this chapter we will discuss:

- what osteoporosis is;

- how common the problem is;

- how osteoporosis is diagnosed;

- how bone is normally made and how it is broken down; and

- the factors that are important in influencing bone changes.

Introduction

The existence of osteoporosis has been known since the times of the Ancient Egyptians. Egyptian mummies of mature men of high status from around 220 BC have been found to have evidence of both osteoarthritis and osteoporosis.

A French pathologist, Jean Lobstein (1777–1835), first described the rare brittle bone disease *osteogenesis imperfecta* but also described bone thinning occurring without this congenital abnormality.

Sir Astley Cooper (1767–1841), a London surgeon with an interest in orthopaedics, was the first to use the term 'osteoporosis'. But the term osteoporosis did not make its way truly into medical terminology until the twentieth century.

Fuller Albright (1900–1969), an American physician with a specialist interest in the metabolism of the human body, established the link with bone loss occurring in women after the menopause.

In 1994 the World Health Organization defined osteoporosis based on the new method of identification of osteoporosis by scanning. However, we have become more aware of the true definition of osteoporosis in recent years as a disease of bone thinning with an increased risk of fracture. It is this increased fracture risk that is the important feature of bone thinning and it is this fracture risk that we seek to decrease.

What is osteoporosis?

Osteoporosis is a bone disease characterized by low bone mass (thin bone) and micro-architectural deterioration of bone tissue (fragile bone), with a consequent increase in bone fragility and therefore risk of fracture.

This is the standard definition used by healthcare professionals to define osteoporosis. Simply put, it is a condition where bones become thin and where the microscopic structure of the bone is quite fragile and, therefore, there is an increased risk of breaks to the bone compared to bone not affected by osteoporosis.

Osteoporosis is a condition where multiple mechanisms come together to cause loss of bone mass and deterioration of the skeletal structure. These factors, together with an increased risk of falls in some people, contribute to the high incidence of fragility fractures in osteoporotic patients.

Osteoporosis is a silent condition with no associated signs or symptoms until fractures occur. Population surveys indicate that fracture rates increase with age and broken bones are particularly common in women.

Fracture can occur in any bone but there are three sites classically associated with osteoporotic fracture: hip (fracture neck of femur); spine (vertebral fractures); and wrist (Colles' fracture) (Table 1.1). These three sites are particularly affected

Table 1.1 Common sites of osteoporotic fracture

Wrist/forearm
Vertebral bodies (spine)
Hip (neck of femur)

by osteoporosis due to the type of bone that they contain. This type of bone (trabecular bone) consists of a thin network of interconnecting bars and plates, which results in a large surface area. Changes at this large surface area influence the bone thickness. Fracture causes pain and can result in disability.

The economic costs of osteoporosis are largely those of hip-fracture costs and is estimated to cost the UK exchequer over £1.7 billion per year.

How common is osteoporosis?

Around 50 000 wrist fractures, 50 000 hip fractures, and 40 000 clinical vertebral fractures are diagnosed every year in the UK (Table 1.2). It is estimated that 10 million Americans over 50 years of age have osteoporosis and that 1.5 million fractures due to osteoporosis occur every year in the USA. It is thought that 1% of women over 60 years and 0.5% of men suffer a vertebral fracture every year. Vertebral fractures are painful and the fracture can lead to loss of height of the sufferer. A kyphosis (curvature of the spine) may also develop. Around half of all vertebral fractures do not present to the medical profession. This may be because some fractures do not cause pain but it is more likely to be because there is an acceptance that back pain is a normal part of ageing. It is, therefore, estimated that around 80 000 vertebral fractures occur in the UK each year.

Hip fractures increase with age, as does the increased risk of death following the fracture.

Many young people suffer fractures but these are mainly fractures of the long bones (arms and legs), and they tend to occur after a traumatic event.

Table 1.2 How common is osteoporosis?

Women	Men
1 in 2 women over the age of 50 years will suffer an osteoporotic fracture.	1 in 5 men over the age of 50 years will suffer an osteoporotic fracture.

They are also more common in men than women—directly opposite to the situation with osteoporotic fractures.

Bone and the skeleton

The adult human skeleton comprises 213 bones, each of which is sculpted by a process called 'modelling' and constantly renewed by a process termed 'remodelling'. The skeleton has three main functions:

- support and movement;

- protection of vital organs; and

- to maintain mineral balance.

Remodelling provides a key role in mineral metabolism and also provides a mechanism for preserving bone strength by replacing older bone with new mechanically sound bone. Mineral metabolism is the mechanism by which certain minerals, such as calcium, magnesium and phosphate are kept in balance in the body.

The composition of bone enables it to perform its unique mechanical, protective, and metabolic functions. Bone consists of:

- minerals (50–70%);

- organic (protein) matrix (20–40%);

- water (5–10%); and

- fats (3%).

The minerals provide the mechanical rigidity and load-bearing strength to the bone. The bone acts as a reservoir for the minerals: calcium, phosphate, and magnesium. The organic matrix (protein component) provides elasticity and flexibility to bone and determines its structural organization. The cells responsible for bone formation, repair, and remodelling respond to hormonal, mechanical, and other outside influences, such as pressure or injury. Fats control the flux of ions, whilst water is important for the maintenance of the tissue and its overall health.

A long bone consists of the ends (epiphyses) and a cylindrical tube connecting the two ends (diaphysis). The zone between the ends and the cylindrical tube is termed the metaphysis. The metaphysis is separated from the epiphysis by a layer of cartilage, which is called the growth plate. The growth plate is responsible for the increase in bone length occurring in childhood. The external part of bone is formed of a thick area of calcified tissue called cortical bone (cortex). At the ends of the bone this encloses a cavity, called the medullary cavity, which contains bone marrow. The cortex becomes thinner towards the middle of the bone and the internal space here is filled with a network of thin calcified bars and plates of bone termed trabecular bone. The spaces between the trabecular bone plates are filled with bone marrow (Fig. 1.1).

Cortical bone fulfils a mainly mechanical and protective function, whilst trabecular bone has a predominately metabolic function. Cortical bone is, therefore, found mainly in long-bone shafts, while trabecular bone (cancellous bone) predominates in spinal bone (vertebrae), ends of bone, and in the ribs. Approximately 85% of bone is cortical.

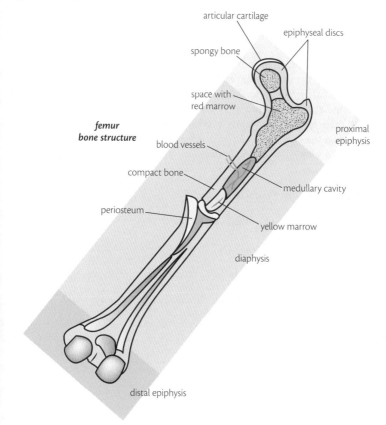

Fig. 1.1 The structure of bone.

Trabecular bone contributes 15% to the total bone mass but, because of its anatomy of interconnecting bars and plates, it has a large surface area and is hence more markedly affected by changes in bone due to ageing or the menopause.

Bone cells

There are three main cells within bone, two of these are involved in making/building bone, and the other is involved in the breakdown of old bone (Table 1.3). The bone-forming cells are:

* osteoblasts: form new bone and produce the bone structure;

* osteocytes: occur throughout the bone, supporting the bone structure and important regulators of bone function.

Osteoblast

The factors involved in making a mature or adult osteoblast have not been fully identified, but many are genetically regulated. Mature osteoblasts are square-shaped cells that have a single nucleus (control centre) and well-developed internal metabolism equipment. They have the ability to make the proteins of the cell matrix, such as collagen, and are metabolically very active cells. They also contain the enzyme alkaline phosphatase, which probably has an important role to play in bone mineralization, although its exact mechanism of action is unknown.

The functions of the osteoblast are to:

* produce the proteins of the bone structure;

* secrete some of the growth factors that are stored in the bone matrix;

* mineralize the newly formed bone structure;

* have a controlling role over bone breakdown cells (osteoclasts).

Table 1.3 The bone cells

Osteoblasts
Osteocytes
Osteoclasts

Many factors stimulate bone and it appears that the osteoblast is the cell that is influenced by these factors (perhaps along with the osteocytes). The osteoblast then further influences other cells, such as the bone-resorbing cells (osteoclasts). The osteoblast, therefore, has a controlling function in bone turnover.

Osteocyte

An osteocyte is an osteoblast, once it has become encased in the bone matrix that it produced. The osteocyte develops numerous connections with adjacent cells to ensure their continued health. All osteocytes are located in spaces (lacunae) and the cellular connections lie in tunnels (canaliculi). The function of the osteocyte is still being finalized but they produce growth hormones and several bone structure proteins. The osteocyte is finally broken down and digested, along with other components of bone, during bone breakdown.

Osteoclasts

Osteoclasts are unique, highly specialized cells, which arise from the bone marrow. Young osteoclasts circulate in the blood and can move to sites where bone resorption (breakdown) is required.

Mature osteoclasts are found on the bone surfaces. They are usually found in contact with a calcified bone surface and within Howship's lacunae (pits in the bone) that are the result of the osteoclasts own bone breakdown activity. They are large cells with numerous nuclei (control centres). There is abundant metabolic apparatus within the osteoclast.

The osteoclasts have a specific area of their cell surface known as the ruffled border, which sits against the bone surface. This area is composed of folds and invaginations that allow intimate contact with the bone surface and is the site of bone breakdown.

Osteoclasts break down bone by the production of enzymes (TRACP and Cathepsin K), which are transported in little balloons and secreted through the ruffled border. Osteoclasts also produce acid and work by dissolving the bone crystals and digesting the collagen fibres. The cell ingests the bone components and then the digested components are released. This explains why bone breakdown helps maintain blood calcium and phosphate levels. At the end of a bone breakdown cycle, the osteoclast dies. The process of normal cell death is sometimes called apoptosis.

Control of bone remodelling

Bone remodelling is a complex process coordinating the breakdown of old bone and formation of new bone. It involves a number of cellular structures that are regulated by hormones and local factors. These hormones and local factors particularly affect osteoblasts and osteoclasts.

Many hormones are involved in this process, such as parathyroid hormone (PTH), vitamin D, oestrogen, and steroids.

Calcitonin

This hormone is secreted by the thyroid gland (thyroidal C-cells). Its synthesis and secretion is under the control of blood calcium levels. Calcitonin is destroyed by the kidney and liver. Calcitonin affects osteoclast function and reduces bone breakdown.

Vitamin D

Vitamin D is made in the skin by the action of sunlight. It is biologically inactive at this stage and undergoes two successive chemical reactions in the liver and kidney to become the biologically active form of vitamin D. The main biological effect of active vitamin D is to maintain the blood calcium within the normal range. This is achieved by increasing the gut absorption of calcium. The kidney production of active vitamin D is tightly regulated by blood calcium levels through the actions of parathyroid hormone and phosphate.

During exposure to sunlight a cholesterol-like agent present in the skin absorbs solar radiation, which in turn causes the transformation of this agent to an early form of vitamin D. This early vitamin D then moves from the skin to the circulation.

The early vitamin D is transported to the liver, where an enzymatic reaction occurs to transform it further. This then enters the circulation and is the main circulating form of vitamin D; it is the most reliable indicator of vitamin D status and is used to determine if people have enough vitamin D stores. This vitamin D is then transported to the kidney where it is further changed, this time into active vitamin D (Fig. 1.2).

In the presence of adequate vitamin D, 30% of dietary calcium and 70% dietary phosphate are absorbed. If vitamin D is low, only 10–15% of the dietary calcium and 60% of dietary phosphate is absorbed. During pregnancy and

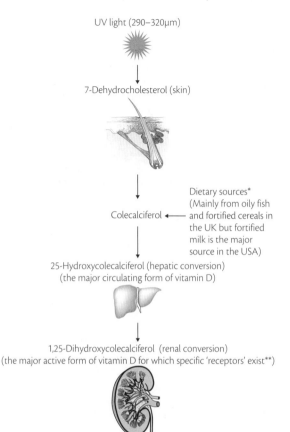

UV light (290–320µm)

7-Dehydrocholesterol (skin)

Colecalciferol ◄——— Dietary sources*
(Mainly from oily fish and fortified cereals in the UK but fortified milk is the major source in the USA)

25-Hydroxycolecalciferol (hepatic conversion)
(the major circulating form of vitamin D)

1,25-Dihydroxycolecalciferol (renal conversion)
(the major active form of vitamin D for which specific 'receptors' exist**)

*As little as 10% of total colecalciferol may be derived from dietary sources
**Specific DNA vitamin D response elements

Fig. 1.2 The generation of bioactive vitamin D *in vivo*.

breast-feeding, an increase in vitamin D, made by the placenta, results in increased gut absorption to 50–80% of the available calcium.

Melanin, which causes skin pigmentation, competes for sunlight and reduces the production of vitamin D. Therefore, different skin colours require differing sunlight exposures to produce the same amount of vitamin D. Ageing also decreases the amount of vitamin D in the skin. For those greater than 70 years of age, less than 30% of vitamin D is produced for the same sunlight exposure as a young adult. Latitude (how far from the equator we live), time of day, and season of year all dramatically affect the production of vitamin D by the skin. Sunlight exposure provides over 80% of our vitamin D requirements. In the United Kingdom, the wavelength of ultraviolet light from the sun is only sufficient to produce vitamin D in the summer months and hence we need to build up our reserves over the summer. When vitamin D production is in excess of current requirements, it can be stored in fat to be used in the winter months. Use of sunscreens (with a sun protection factor above 8) will substantially reduce the skin production of vitamin D by more than 97%.

Foodstuffs provide little of our vitamin D requirements. Oily fish, fish oils, and egg yolks are the only common sources of vitamin D in food. In some countries (such as the USA), certain food groups are fortified with vitamin D.

Parathyroid hormone (PTH)

PTH and the active form of vitamin D are the principle regulators of calcium in humans. In bone, PTH causes the release of calcium and phosphate. This leads to an increase in blood calcium levels and a decrease in blood phosphate levels. Parathyroid hormone is produced in the parathyroid glands, which sit behind the thyroid gland. There are usually four parathyroid glands (Fig. 1.3).

The effects of PTH on bone depend on the presence of osteoblasts and osteoclasts. The osteoblast has a central role in directing the actions of PTH. PTH causes bone breakdown by its effects on osteoclasts. PTH increases bone formation by its effects on osteoblasts.

PTH secretion occurs episodically in normal subjects with small peaks of the hormone occurring several times a day, each lasting for several minutes.

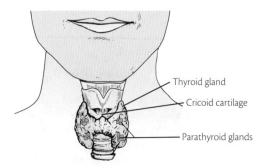

Thyroid gland

Cricoid cartilage

Parathyroid glands

Fig. 1.3 The parathyroid glands.

Additionally PTH is secreted in a 24-hour rhythm, with an early morning peak and mid-afternoon low levels.

The bone matrix

The bone matrix (structure) is made up of lots of proteins, of which collagen is the most important.

Collagen

Type 1 collagen is the basic building block of the bone matrix. Bone collagen is the most important and abundant protein, with 90% in the form of type 1 collagen. Type 1 collagen is a highly coiled structure. It is insoluble. When collagen molecules are broken down, this leads to the formation of small fragments of collagen. Measurement of these small fragments has proved to be a valuable measurement of bone breakdown.

Non-collagen proteins

Non-collagen proteins account for 10–15% of the total protein content. Four types of non-collagen protein exist: proteoglycans, growth-related proteins, cell attachment proteins, and carboxylated Gla proteins.

The physiological roles for individual bone protein constituents are not well-defined. However, they may help not only in regulating bone but also in the control of osteoblast and osteoclast metabolism.

Bone remodelling

Coupling of bone turnover

In normal conditions, bone formation and bone breakdown work in cooperation and in balance; this is termed bone coupling. Packets of bone that are removed during bone breakdown are replaced during bone formation (Fig. 1.4).

All diseases of bone are superimposed on the normal remodelling process. Progressive bone loss after age 40 years, depending on the bone, occurs in all humans and indicates an imbalance between bone breakdown and bone formation.

The regulation of bone turnover is complex but the understanding of this is leading to a true understanding of why osteoporosis occurs and is providing mechanisms that can be targeted to prevent bone thinning.

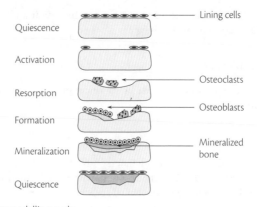

Fig. 1.4 The remodelling cycle.

The concept that the stimulation of bone breakdown requires the interaction between osteoblast and osteoclast cells was put forward many years ago, but the actual mechanism for this was only discovered recently. Osteoblasts produce compounds called RANKL and osteoprotegerin (OPG). These two compounds have opposite effects on bone breakdown. RANKL binds to its receptor (RANK) on osteoclasts and causes bone breakdown. OPG can block this effect by acting as a 'dummy' blocker of the receptor

Bone changes throughout life

During childhood there is a steady increase in bone thickness, accompanying the increased length of bone as a child ages and grows. Puberty greatly increases height and also bone thickness. At the end of puberty, final height-attainment occurs and the growth plates in bone fuse. Extra bone thickness can still be acquired, although at a lower rate than during puberty. Final peak bone mass is achieved during the third decade of life, i.e. between the ages of 20 and 30 (Fig. 1.5). This peak bone thickness is largely genetically determined, with 75% of the bone mass being the result of genetic influences. Diet, exercise, and health issues largely account for the other fluctuations in peak bone mass. It is recognized that race also affects the peak bone thickness with the Black population having higher bone mass than those of the Caucasian and Asian communities. Males also achieve a higher peak bone mass than females. During mid-adult life, bone mass is remarkably constant but again can be adversely affected by factors such as smoking and alcohol intake, and by many medical conditions, which will be discussed in Chapter 2. The menopause brings a period of rapid bone loss to women and old age brings further gradual bone loss, with the added risk of an increasing tendency to fall.

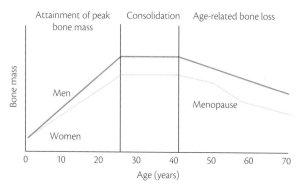

Fig. 1.5 Changes in bone mass during life.

➡ Summary

Much is now known of the underlying biological mechanisms that result in bone strength development and the reasons for bone thinning. The understanding of bone biology is leading to a greater awareness of those at potential risk of bone thinning, and also provides a means to develop medications to reduce the burden of osteoporosis. We also recognize that bone thickness itself is not the only factor that is important in fractures, equally important is the individual's risk of falling. Prevention of falls and maintaining good general health is also essential in the prevention of fractures.

2

Who gets osteoporosis?

➜ Key points

- Bone thickness changes throughout life.

- Genetic factors account for up to 75% of our maximum bone strength.

- Smoking and excess intake of alcohol have a negative impact on bone health.

- A good calcium and vitamin D intake is essential for bone health.

- Weight-bearing exercise encourages the development of strong bones and exercise reduces falls risks.

- Many medications and diseases can influence our bone thickness.

In this chapter we will discuss those who would be considered at increased risk of developing osteoporosis, and the reasons for this increased risk.

Introduction

Bone is a living structure, like our hair and nails and skin it grows and is broken down constantly throughout life. The thickness of our bone at any point in our life is due to everything that has had an influence on our bone up until that time point.

Some of these factors we can influence/change, some are inherent characteristics that we cannot alter. Generally our bones build up to peak by our third decade, stay stable for a period, and then we all lose a little bone from our fifth decade onwards. Women additionally have a period of more rapid bone loss at the menopause.

Post-menopausal osteoporosis in women occurs when the bone mass falls to a level where fracture risks are increased. That critical bone mass level is the result of the woman's peak bone mass achievement and how much bone she loses later in life, along, of course, with the severity of any injury or fall sustained (see below).

In men, without menopausal bone loss, there is more likely to be an alternative or secondary cause of low bone density (such as steroid therapy or alcohol excess) present in their medical history.

Where it all begins: the genetics of osteoporosis

It has been estimated that 75% of our maximum achievable bone strength, called our peak bone mass, is genetically determined. Also, later in life bone loss may be influenced by genetic factors. Many candidate genes have been considered in previous research, such as the vitamin D receptor gene, the oestrogen receptor gene, and the collagen type 1α1 gene. Genetic effects on the skeleton are likely to be due to many genes acting in tandem.

Information on the genetic importance of defining our risk of osteoporosis derive from studies on twins or close family members with the disease, or by studying single gene mutations in populations by candidate gene studies, or by a widespread search of the human genome.

The importance of genetic factors is illustrated by the results of twin and family studies, which indicate that heredity accounts for between 50 and 85% of the variation in bone mineral density, depending on the specific skeletal site examined. To date, only around 20% of the total variation in bone mineral density (BMD) at attainment of peak bone mass can be accounted for by the genetic variations already known. Both bone mineral density and fracture risk appear to be inherited, and lots of different genes seem to be involved in the process. Genetic research is a rapidly expanding area in the bone field.

Peak bone mass

Peak bone mass is the maximum bone mass achieved in the third decade of life. It is influenced by many factors, the most influential being that of genetic variation. There are also many environmental factors that influence BMD and peak bone mass achievement, and these probably interact with genetic elements (Table 2.1).

Table 2.1 Important factors in bone health

Genetics
Diet
Exercise
Smoking
Alcohol
Hormonal deficiency
Medical illnesses and medications

Weight-bearing exercise in childhood and adolescence positively increases bone thickness. Many studies of exercise in childhood have demonstrated great gains in bone mass. It is, however, essential to continue the exercise intervention long-term for sustained improvements to occur.

Nutritional factors are well-recognized determinants of peak bone mass, particularly calcium intake. Children have a greater requirement for a good calcium intake than adults and there are concerns that our modern diet has reduced milk consumption in children who, therefore, have a poorer calcium intake than desirable.

Conditions resulting in malabsorption of foods, such as coeliac disease and cystic fibrosis, have adverse effects on bone. In a child with cystic fibrosis there are the additional affects of chronic infection and low body weight, with their negative impacts on bone health.

Anorexia nervosa, where the individual female affected often stops menstruating for a time (referred to as periods of amenorrhoea), as well as being nutritionally deprived also poses an additional risk of bone thinning or loss. Other conditions that result in amenorrhoea, such as primary ovarian failure, excessive exercise, and pituitary gland abnormalities, all have detrimental effects on BMD.

Smoking and excessive alcohol intake adversely affects peak bone mass attainment. Caffeine may also have a negative role. Although there is no evidence that fizzy drinks are bad for bone, where they are drunk instead of milk, they will have a negative effect on the overall calcium intake.

Case study

A 12-year-old girl slipped and fell in the playground at school and has severe back pain. Her general practitioner quickly referred her for some X-rays because of pre-existing problems with her general health. The X-rays showed that she had suffered three vertebral fractures.

This 12-year-old had been undergoing treatment over the previous 9 months for a rare liver tumour. Her treatment had involved radiotherapy, chemotherapy, and then surgical removal of the tumour.

During her chemotherapy she received high doses of oral steroid medications. She was referred for a dual energy X-ray absorptiometry (DXA) scan, and she and her mother attended together. Both were naturally worried about the nature of the scan she was about to have but relieved to find it such a simple, painless, and quick procedure. She was found to have very low bone density for her age on DXA scanning.

Advice was given by the bone unit to her paediatrician who started treatment. This treatment was in the form of a bisphosphonate medicine, given, in this case, into a vein (i.e. intravenous rather than orally, as more scientific evidence exists to support this treatment in children). After 1 year she had a repeat scan performed and excellent improvements in her bone mass were seen. Further treatment was not required and she has experienced no further fractures in 6 years of follow-up and remains well with no recurrence of her liver tumour.

Dietary factors in bone health

Dietary factors appear to influence bone metabolism. There is evidence that calcium, magnesium, zinc, vitamin C, and other nutrients associated with fruit and vegetable intake, and both protein intake and overall energy intake, influence bone metabolism. However, is not known in what way such nutrients affect bone turnover; they may be markers for other factors affecting bone health. Studies of short-term changes in dietary protein intake have suggested that this leads to a decrease in absorption of calcium from the gut. However, diets high in protein, when they occur in the setting of a good calcium intake, may be beneficial in preventing fractures in the elderly. Perhaps high protein intakes are simply a reflection of good general health and adequate monetary income. Low-salt diets appear to reduce the amount of calcium that is lost by the kidney and, therefore, may have a positive effect on bone thickness.

Smoking

Smoking status is known to effect bone turnover and there is some suggestion from small studies that this is due to the suppression of the PTH–vitamin D endocrine system. The gut absorption rates of calcium in smokers have been found to be lower, as have serum calcium and PTH concentrations. Smoking has been found to increase fracture rates in older men. It is also recognized that female smokers tend to have an earlier menopause than non-smokers.

Loss of oestrogen secretion at the menopause

From the fourth decade onwards there is a gradual loss of bone mass occurring at a rate of <1% per year. In men, this rate of loss continues throughout the remainder of their lives. In women, decreased oestrogen, occurring in the peri-menopausal and immediate post-menopausal years, results in increased bone loses of around 2% per year. Marked individual variations occur in this bone loss, with some women losing higher rates of bone and/or over a longer period of time. By the time of the seventh decade, the bone loss slows again to around <1% per year and continues at this rate. Over her lifetime a woman will lose, on average, 30–40% of her peak bone mass.

📄 Case study

A 73-year-old lady, normally fit and well, living independently in her own home, fell at home and broke her right hip. The fracture liaison service referred her automatically to have a bone density scan, once she had recovered sufficiently to have the scan in comfort.

The DXA scan revealed severe osteoporosis. She was seen at a metabolic bone disease clinic and on questioning was found to have a history of an early menopause, aged 37, with no hormone replacement therapy treatment.

She was given an oral bisphosphonate tablet to be taken weekly and, additionally, given a calcium and vitamin D supplement. An osteoporosis specialist nurse spent time with her explaining the diagnosis and giving information to help prevent future falls.

Other influences on bone mass and fracture risk

Other factors have additional negative effects on bone density and fracture risk, such as lack of vitamin D exposure, poor general health, poor mobility, and poor vision. Most of these factors increase fracture risk by increasing the risk of falls. The two most important determinants of an individual's risk of fracture are their bone thickness and their age.

Male osteoporosis

It is estimated that around 1 in 5 men sustain fractures related to osteoporosis. Peak bone mass is achieved in the same general timeframe as in women and also with the same general determinants. The peak attainment occurs a little later and is slightly higher than in women. A less than 1% per year decrease in bone mass occurs from the start of the fifth decade onwards but this level of loss is maintained throughout the subsequent decades. Far fewer studies of male bone loss have been conducted.

Male osteoporosis is more likely to occur as the result of a secondary cause of osteoporosis, such as malabsorption of food, steroid therapy, or alcohol excess, than would be expected in women, due to the lack of a distinct menopause in men. Around 30–50% of men with osteoporosis have a recognized secondary cause.

Testosterone deficiency is a major aetiological factor in up to 30% of men presenting with spinal osteoporosis and there is some evidence to implicate oestrogen deficiency also in the causation of male osteoporosis.

Oestrogen is essential for normal bone development in young men; oestrogen concentrations also affect bone remodelling, bone density, and rates of bone loss in older men, more strongly than do testosterone levels.

📄 Case study

A 69-year-old male smoker suffered a simple fall, when he tripped on a kerb stone. This led to a fractured of his upper arm. As part of the fracture liaison service, he was automatically referred for a DXA scan. This DXA scan revealed very thin bones for his age and sex.

Mr X had a past history of smoking and also of a heavy alcohol intake whilst he was working abroad. He was very surprised to find that his bones were thin, as he thought that osteoporosis only affected women. He was also concerned to realize the significance of his previous smoking and alcohol excess.

Mr X was given an oral weekly bisphosphonate tablet with two calcium and vitamin D supplements to take every day. He found these quite easy to take, which surprised him as he was not used to taking any other tablets or medicines.

General lifestyle advice regarding particularly diet, alcohol intake, and smoking was also given. Three years later he had a follow up DXA scan, which revealed some improvements in his bone thickness and, most importantly, he has not had any further bone fractures.

Secondary causes of osteoporosis

Some medical conditions are associated with osteoporosis as part of their overall disease complex. It is essential to identify these conditions when investigating and subsequently managing a patient with osteoporosis, in order to improve the overall prognosis (Table 2.2). Also, knowledge that such conditions are associated with osteoporosis can allow targeting of osteoporosis services towards these high-risk individuals (Table 2.3).

Table 2.2 Routine laboratory tests used to exclude/identify secondary causes of osteoporosis

Biochemical blood tests	Tests of: kidney, bone, and liver function. Tests of vitamin D levels
Haematological blood tests	Full blood count and erythrocyte sedimentation rate (reflection of body inflammation).
Endocrinological blood tests	Tests of: thyroid function, sex hormone levels, and antibody test for coeliac disease.

📄 Case study

A 42-year-old woman, Ms A had recently experienced symptoms of the menopause (hot flushes, irregular periods, and irritability). Her general practitioner sent her for a DXA scan to help her decide whether hormone replacement therapy would be a valuable treatment for her.

Her DXA scan revealed marked osteoporosis, particularly for her age.

As the result was unexpectedly low, she was referred to the local metabolic bone disease clinic. There a thorough history was taken and it appeared that she had suffered recurrent episodes of iron-deficiency anaemia and for many years had been of low body weight.

Blood tests performed at the clinic suggested she might be suffering from coeliac disease. In this condition there is an allergy to gluten (a part of wheat), which results in very poor absorption of food from the small bowel.

After confirmatory tests by the gastroenterologists, she was given a gluten-free diet, calcium and vitamin D supplements, and also hormone replacement therapy. Very quickly she felt much better within herself with more energy and she put on a little weight.

Good improvements were also seen in her bone mass over the next 5 years and in her longer-term general health.

Table 2.3 Secondary causes of osteoporosis

Bone cancers	Myeloma
	Primary bone cancer
	Secondary bone cancer
Endocrine causes	Overactive thyroid gland
	Overproduction of steroids
	Low sex hormone levels
	Under- and overactive parathyroid glands
	Pituitary problems
Renal disease	Chronic kidney failure

(continued)

Table 2.3 Secondary causes of osteoporosis *(continued)*

Gastrointestinal disease	Gastrectomy (removal of stomach)
	Malabsorption
	Chronic liver disease including cirrhosis
Other hereditary bone and connective tissue diseases	Osteogenesis imperfecta
	Marfan's syndrome
	Ehlers–Danlos
	Homocysenuria
Medications	Heparin
	Corticosteroids
	Aromatase Inhibitors used to treat breast cancer
Miscellaneous	Anorexia nervosa
	Chronic alcoholism
	Immobilization
	Rheumatoid arthritis and other inflammatory arthritis problems

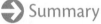 Summary

Whilst osteoporosis is a common occurrence with ageing there are medical conditions that can predispose to bone thinning at an earlier age. Understanding of those at special risks has led many specialty organizations, such as the British Thoracic Society, the Society of Gastroenterologists, and the Endocrine Society, to issue specific guidance on those patients at increased risk of the future development of osteoporosis.

3

The diagnosis of osteoporosis

➲ Key points

◆ The World Health Organization (WHO) developed criteria for the diagnosis of osteoporosis in post-menopausal women in 1994.

◆ DXA scanning is the gold standard diagnostic test.

◆ X-rays are important in the identification of fractures.

◆ Blood tests for 'biochemical markers of bone turnover' are now available to provide a measurement of bone change.

◆ Bone biopsies provide additional valuable information.

Introduction

This chapter will discuss the techniques available for the diagnosis and assessment of the extent of bone thinning and its response to treatment.

The WHO definition of osteoporosis was formulated in 1994 and is based on bone mineral density (BMD) as measured by dual energy X-ray absorptiometry (DXA) scanning. The term osteoporosis is applied when the individual's BMD, at either hip or spine site, is less than 2.5 standard deviations (SDs) below the sex-specific young adult mean BMD. These SDs are termed T scores (Table 3.1).

The T-score cut-off of –2.5 was selected in 1994 so that the proportion of patients identified as having osteoporosis would equate to the known lifetime risk of osteoporotic fracture. This T-score figure has proven to be a very helpful cut-off to categorize an individual's future and current risk of fracture.

Table 3.1 World Health Organization (WHO) definitions of osteoporosis and T-score classification of BMD in women

T-score	Interpretation
$T \leq -2.5$	Osteoporosis—the BMD result is equal to, or more than, 2.5 SDs below the young adult mean BMD
$T \leq -1$ but is > -2.5	Osteopaenia—the BMD result is between 1 and 2.5 SDs below the young adult mean BMD
$T > -1$	Normal—the BMD result is less than 1 SD below the young adult mean BMD

Other factors are important too, however, such as age, weight, and the presence of other risk factors for osteoporosis, including diseases causing increases in bone turnover, such as an overactive thyroid gland and steroid therapy. Quantifying an individual's risk of future fracture is an important part of the osteoporosis assessment, and guides the need for therapies for osteoporosis. This could be considered as being similar to the decisions used to treat people with high blood pressure or high cholesterol levels, to reduce the future risk of a heart attack or stroke.

X-rays

Prior to specific scanning procedures X-ray evidence was used to suggest low bone mass. Unfortunately around 30% of bone mass must be lost before simple X-ray visualization will identify thinning bone and quantifying this loss was impossible. Today the role of X-rays is the detection of fractures, particularly vertebral fractures. Spinal X-rays also allow measurement of the severity of fractures and can help exclude other aetiologies for fracture, such as myeloma (a specific type of bone cancer) and other bone malignancy.

Finally, spinal X-rays can provide a supporting role in the reporting of DXA scans, since fractures, osteoarthritis, and other vertebral deformities can give falsely elevated BMD results by DXA scanning (Fig. 3.1).

Dual energy X-ray absorptiometry

Dual energy X-ray absorptiometry (DXA) is a precise and a relatively inexpensive technology. An X-ray tube provides the photons and the dual effect is achieved by alternating the voltage across the X-ray tube. The radiation exposure for a standard hip and spine scan is very low and is less than 10% of a

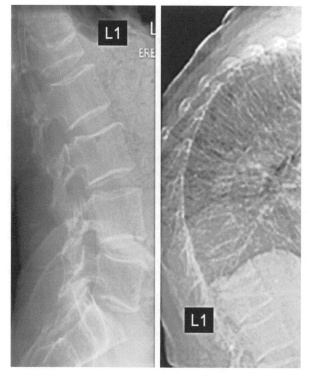

Fig. 3.1 Thoraco-lumbar spine X-rays showing vertebral fractures.

departmental chest X-ray. This is roughly the equivalent of standard back-ground radiation, and less than background radiation in Aberdeen or Dartmoor, for example. The higher resolution of newer DXA machines has meant that images, particularly of the lateral spine, can now be assessed for vertebral size and shape, which allows identification of vertebral fractures in many cases without the widespread use of higher radiation spinal X-rays.

Three main manufacturers make DXA scanners: Hologic, GE Lunar, and Norland. None of the scans from the different machines can be directly com-pared to each other, but should give overall similar results. The diagnostic criteria for osteoporosis, set up by the WHO in 1994, are based on DXA scanning. DXA scanning can also be used to monitor improvements in bone density with therapy. DXA scanning is currently the 'gold standard' in the diagnosis of osteoporosis.

The precision (reproducibility of the result) of a spinal scan is between 1 and 2%, while that of a hip scan is 3–5%. This is extremely good for a piece of medical equipment but does mean that an interval of 2 years is required before changes in the DXA scan result can be considered as a reliable indicator of actual changes in BMD at the spine, either due to bone loss or due to increase in bone due to treatment. In the hip area, a re-scan interval of 3–5 years is required before the scan change is a reliable indicator of actual BMD change in the individual patient (Table 3.2).

Of great importance in DXA scanning is the positioning of the patient and the areas of interest, the scan analysis, and knowledge of factors that might interfere with the scan result (i.e. a recent barium enema, osteoarthritis in the spine, or a piercing ring). The National Osteoporosis Society in the UK runs courses to enable radiographers to acquire specialist knowledge and qualification in DXA scanning. The gold standard scan is one performed by an accredited specialist radiographer, checked by a trained medical specialist and reported by a trained physician in the bone field (Fig. 3.2).

Peripheral bone density machines exist but should be considered largely as screening tools only, not as diagnostic instruments. Monitoring change is not possible using a peripheral DXA device.

Quantitative computerized tomography

Quantitative computerized tomography (QCT) can be adapted to quantify bone mineral content at the spine. The method has a high reproducibility but is a sophisticated and demanding technique. It is expensive, time-consuming, and uses more radiation than other methods of bone density assessment. Therefore, QCT is not useful in the monitoring of change in bone density over time. The main advantage is that it can separate out the different types of bone in the scanning procedure. This presently has little benefit to the individual patient but is useful in the research field. Forearm and hip QCT are also used in research settings.

Table 3.2 DXA scanning

Low-dosage radiation technique
Accurate assessment
Reproducible result
Non-invasive and not claustrophobic

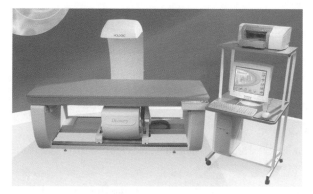

Fig. 3.2 A modern axial (hip and spine) DXA scanner.

Peripheral ultrasound

Ultrasound scanners have been developed to look at peripheral bone density, particularly of the heal site. Studies have shown that this portable non-radiation-using technique can be valuable at predicting risk of future hip fracture, particularly in the elderly, and it may have a future role in screening for osteoporosis. Ultrasound does not measure the true thickness of the bone but potentially provides some measurement of the integrity of the bone. If some-one has an ultrasound scan that suggests bone thinning, a DXA scan would be indicated to confirm or refute the findings.

Biochemical markers of bone turnover

The improved understanding of the function of bone cells, their physiology, and the physiology of bone has allowed the development in recent years of biochemical markers, measured in blood and urine, which reflect the relative activity of bone formation and bone breakdown. These biochemical methods have enhanced our understanding of bone turnover in many different areas and have provided a non-invasive method of obtaining information on the changes in bone without the requirement for a bone biopsy. This has been of great value in the area of bone research but these markers are also becoming established in clinical practice for monitoring response and compliance to medications. Additionally, it is now established that high bone turnover itself is an additional risk factor for fracture, over and above the bone density.

Bone markers, therefore, provide a dynamic measurement of bone turnover, whilst a measurement of bone mineral density is a static measure of bone thickness at that moment in time.

Bone formation markers

Alkaline phosphatase

Alkaline phosphatase is an enzyme made by the liver, bone, kidney, and placenta. The enzyme plays a key role in bone mineralization. A specific test now exists to pick up the bone form of the enzyme only and this has provided the basis for a specific measure of bone formation—bone-specific alkaline phosphatase (BSAP).

Osteocalcin

Bone-forming cells produce a hormone called osteocalcin. Measuring osteocalcin reflects bone formation.

Propeptide extension peptides of type 1 collagen (P1CP and P1NP)

When the collagen molecules of bone are being made, small parts of the collagen are broken off and can be measured in blood.

Bone breakdown markers

Pyridinoline crosslinks and crosslinked C and N telopeptides

When bone is broken down, small parts of the collagen molecules are released and can be measured in blood and urine. They are influenced by diet and by time of day, so are best checked in fasted people, first thing in the morning.

High bone turnover is found in the elderly with low vitamin D, both those living in nursing homes and the free-living elderly. It has been shown that markers of bone breakdown predict hip fracture in elderly women, independent of the bone density of these women. This suggests that the combination of BMD measurement with a bone breakdown marker could be a better predictor of hip fracture risk in the elderly.

Bone markers can also be used to monitor the effects of therapies such as HRT and bisphosphonates. It may, therefore, in the future be possible for bone markers to:

- help predict risk of fracture;

- select patients for treatment;

- select treatments for patients;

- monitor effectiveness of treatments;

- predict response to treatment.

Bone biopsies

Occasionally a bone biopsy is taken from the main bone of the pelvis to look under the microscope at the structure of the bone. The biopsy procedure is done under local anaesthetic, usually in a day-ward facility. Most patients do require some degree of sedation for the procedure but it is generally very well-tolerated. A small wound is left, which is closed using a suture; this will leave a small scar around 1 cm in size.

This is not a standard procedure for all patients, as in most cases enough information can be gathered from DXA scans, X-rays, and blood tests; however, when required it can provide very detailed information. Sometimes, prior to the biopsy, the subject is asked to take a tablet (a specific antibiotic medication) for a few days 2 weeks before the procedure. This tablet is combined into bone and shows up on the biopsy telling the doctor how quickly the bones are being remodelled.

⊃ Summary

The assessment of a person thought to be at risk of osteoporosis requires a good history to be taken of factors such as:

⬥ family history of fracture;

⬥ steroid therapy and other medications;

⬥ medical conditions; and

⬥ previous fracture history.

A DXA scan will usually provide enough information to confirm or refute a diagnosis of osteoporosis. If such a diagnosis is found, the clinician will check blood tests to find other causes of bone thinning, and may also perform some tests to find out how quickly the bones are being made and broken down.

If doubt remained of the diagnosis, or some unusual features were present, a bone biopsy might be performed to help clarify the situation.

4

The management and medical treatments for osteoporosis— now and the future

➲ Key points

◆ Recent advances in bone biology have greatly increased the types of medication now available to treat osteoporosis.

◆ Bisphosphonates are the main treatments and are available as weekly and monthly tablets, as well as by intravenous (IV) injections.

◆ Whilst hormone replacement therapy (HRT) has become a less popular therapy, it still has a very important place, particularly in the younger man or woman.

◆ Parathyroid-like therapies have greatly improved treatment approaches for those with very severe osteoporosis.

◆ Much active research is ongoing to produce new types of medicine to treat osteoporosis.

In this chapter we will deal with the management of osteoporosis and the prevention of fracture; we will also consider some of the new therapies under study.

The management of osteoporosis

Prevention

The prevention of osteoporosis is a very important part of its management. Achievement of a good peak bone mass by increasing weight-bearing exercise in the young and improvements in diet, particularly dietary calcium intake during childhood and adolescence, should reduce the overall burden of osteoporosis. Reduction in smoking, and discouraging excess caffeine and alcohol intakes are also advocated. In the elderly, fall-prevention strategies should be developed in a dual approach to decrease fractures, both by increasing bone strength and decreasing fall frequency. Such approaches should include eyesight tests, safety in the home, and assessments of diuretic and blood pressure tablet use, which could cause dizziness, and considering the issue of hip protectors for the vulnerable. This is discussed in greater detail in other chapters (Table 4.1).

Case study

A 78-year-old woman was seen by her general practitioner after a simple fall where she fractured her wrist. He realized from speaking to her that she fell quite often and had had three falls in the last 6 months alone.

In the past she had broken both her wrists and also her hip after a simple fall.

The GP referred her for a bone density scan at her local hospital. The bone scan showed that her bone density was actually above average for her age. This meant that bone thinning was not the explanation as to why she had suffered the three fractures. Instead her GP felt they were because of her falling.

Mrs M was referred to a falls clinic run in her local hospital to prevent further falling. There she saw a doctor, a physiotherapist, and an occupation therapist. Her medications were checked and she had a general physical examination. The occupational therapist also came to visit her at home to make sure that she was living in safe and suitable accommodation.

She was then seen at a physiotherapy exercise class twice per week for 6 months and her confidence and mobility improved. She also fell far less frequently.

Table 4.1 Prevention of osteoporosis

Exercise
Good calcium intake
Stop smoking
Reduce caffeine intake
Reduce alcohol intake
Fall prevention

Medications for osteoporosis

The aim of the medical management of osteoporosis with drugs is to prevent the consequences of having thin bones, reducing the risk of fracture. Rather like taking blood pressure tablets or cholesterol-lowering medication to reduce the risk of heart disease and stroke, osteoporosis medications have to be taken regularly in an attempt to prevent fracture. They do not make people feel better and hence it is important to ensure that people taking these medications understand the importance of taking their medication long-term, without seeing any immediate apparent benefits from their medication (Table 4.2).

Table 4.2 Management and drug treatment of osteoporosis

Types of medication	Mechanism of action
Bisphosphonates	Oral and intravenous preparations taken fasted, reduce bone breakdown.
HRT	Oral. Patch and gel preparations, reduce bone breakdown.
Selective oestrogen receptor modulators	Oral medications with hormone-like activity, reduce bone breakdown.
PTH analogues	Self-administered daily injections, stimulate bone formation.
Strontium ranelate	Oral sachet mixed with water, taken at night, reduce bone breakdown whilst enhancing bone formation.

Calcium and vitamin D

Calcium and vitamin D supplements in the housebound elderly have been found to decrease hip-fracture risk, probably by reversing the excessive secretion of parathyroid hormone, which occurs when we have inadequate vitamin D stores. There is also evidence of a reduction in the risk of falling, as vitamin D therapy appears to improve lower limb function by increasing muscle strength. It has been estimated from studies that the risk of falls can be reduced by around 20% in older individuals by the use of vitamin D supplements. The optimal amount of vitamin D required for bone health is hotly contested, particularly in the USA where much higher levels are advocated than were previously thought necessary and the amount of vitamin D we obtain from dietary sources, rather than sunlight, are also debated.

Results from a recent large study have indicated that calcium and vitamin D supplements alone do not reduce fracture risk in the elderly living in their own homes.

It is recognized that all patients with osteoporosis, or at risk of osteoporosis, should have a good calcium and vitamin D intake; sometimes this is only achieved by taking calcium and vitamin D supplements. Patients using other medication for osteoporosis do need to have good calcium and vitamin D status.

Recently there has been some controversy about calcium supplements and a potential link with increases in heart disease and stroke. We do not recommend that people supplement their diet with over-the-counter calcium supplements. If dietary calcium intakes are low, then the diet should be enhanced. If this cannot occur by improvements in the diet, a medical practitioner should decide whether calcium and vitamin D supplements will be beneficial.

There is no evidence that calcium and vitamin D supplements in patients with proven osteoporosis increase the risk of cardiovascular disease.

Active bone medications

Pharmaceutical therapies for osteoporosis have traditionally been divided into two types:

- antiresorptive (reducing bone breakdown) and

- anabolic therapies (promoting bone formation).

Recently, the introduction of strontium ranelate to the medication armoury has led to a new addition to these two types of medications. This new group is termed the dual-action bone agents (DABAs). Strontium ranelate is the only

Table 4.3 Therapies for osteoporosis

Antiresorptive agents: reduce bone breakdown	Anabolic agents: enhance bone formation	Dual-action bone agents: reduce bone breakdown whilst also increasing bone formation
HRT	PTH analogues	Strontium ranelate
Bisphosphonates		
Selective oestrogen-receptor antagonists		

current member of this group which may reduce bone breakdown whilst also increasing bone formation. This effect has been best seen in animals and the mechanism of action in humans is less clear-cut.

The medicines available for the management of osteoporosis will be considered under these three headings (Table 4.3).

Antiresorptive agents
Hormone Replacement Therapy (HRT)

Decreasing oestrogen levels at the menopause result in bone loss. Menopause refers to the cessation of menstruation, which occurs around the age of 50 years in most healthy women. The decline in ovarian hormone production is gradual and starts several years before the last period is experienced. Hormone replacement therapy (HRT) given at that time can prevent this bone loss. Many studies have shown that after 3 years of HRT there is around a 20% difference in bone thickness (density) between those taking HRT and those who chose not to take HRT. It has also been shown that prevention of bone loss is possible in all parts of the skeleton with HRT and that HRT reduces the risk of fracture at spine, hip, and peripheral sites.

The effects of oestrogen on the skeleton are complex. However, it is believed that the main action of oestrogen is on the osteoclasts, decreasing bone breakdown.

Table 4.4 Methods of giving HRT

Tablets taken by mouth
Skin patches or gels applied to the skin
Implants under the skin given by a doctor or nurse

The method of taking oestrogen is unimportant. The transdermal (patch) route is as effective as the oral or subcutaneous routes (Table 4.4). Most studies were performed using high oestrogen doses but there is evidence that even lower doses of oestrogen can have beneficial effects. When oestrogen is discontinued, women lose bone at a faster rate than would be expected for the individual's age and at similar rates to those seen within 5 years of the menopause.

The potential side-effects that can occur with HRT have been widely reported in the media. There is an increased risk of endometrial cancer, if oestrogens alone are prescribed. It is, therefore, essential that oestrogen and progesterone be used appropriately together in a woman who has not had a hysterectomy (Table 4.5).

The potential risk of breast cancer with long-term oestrogen therapy has been the adverse event that has most limited the acceptability of long-term HRT. There is little doubt that long-term use of HRT does increase breast cancer risks, although the cancers found tend to be earlier and potentially more readily amenable to treatment.

Further concerns have been raised about heart disease and stroke with HRT therapy. Until recently, accepted wisdom was that HRT had favourable affects on blood lipid (cholesterol and fat) profiles and was beneficial in the prevention of heart disease, and potentially both stroke disease and dementia. However recent studies, such as the Women's Health Initiative (WHI) study using HRT with oestrogen and progestogen given continuously to prevent return of menstruation, have suggested that these assumptions are incorrect. Two large studies have discontinued early due to increased reports of heart problems. Whether these studies pertain only to continuous combined (i.e. oestrogen and progesterone used in a continuous manner rather than in a cyclical fashion) or whether they can be applied to all HRT therapies is unknown. The recently published 'million women' study suggested a gradient of risk from oestrogen alone, through cyclical HRT, and then the continuous combined preparations.

Table 4.5 Types of HRT preparations

Containing oestrogen only
Containing oestrogen and progesterone, with the progesterone used for 7–10 days every month
Oestrogen and progesterone therapy given together on a continuous basis

To further complicate this already confusing area, information from the WHI study in 2007 suggested there had been an exaggeration of the cardiovascular risks, particularly in the younger women, whilst the million women study data has recently reported an increase in ovarian cancer with HRT, which seems independent of the method of delivery of the HRT. This has led to recent guidance to physicians to restrict HRT treatment to those with menopausal symptoms in their 50s and for a maximum interval of around 5 years.

Understandably, with all the adverse publicity, HRT has become unacceptable to many women, but should still be encouraged in those with an early menopause who have an increased risk of future osteoporosis and in whom, at least initially, the increased risk of breast cancer does not apply. It should also be remembered that HRT does reduce the risk of all osteoporotic fractures and appears also to reduce the incidence of bowel cancer.

📄 Case study

Mrs A is a 38-year-old woman who visited her GP complaining of hot flushes and sweats. Her GP performed some bloods tests and confirmed that she was becoming menopausal. Mrs A, 5 years ago, had an overactive thyroid gland. Her GP remembered this and thought it best that she have a bone density scan in case her bones were prematurely thinning.

Her DXA scan revealed slightly thin bones for her age.

The report from the scanning department suggested she took HRT until around the age 50 years or so. Mrs A was not keen on this, as she had read that HRT increased the risk of breast cancer. Her own doctor reassured her but he also asked the menopause clinic at her local hospital to review her.

Mrs A felt that the menopause clinic was very helpful and she particularly benefited from speaking to the menopause specialist nurse. She was commenced on HRT and felt gradually better over the next month. She plans to continue her HRT over the next 10 years.

Bisphosphonates

First reports of the biological effects of bisphosphonates occurred in 1968. Bisphosphonates are compounds of pyrophosphate, which is a naturally occurring compound used as an anti-scaling additive in washing powders and as industrial cleaners. Bisphosphonates are like pyrophosphate but the phosphorus–oxygen (POP) bond is replaced by a phosphorus–carbon (PCP)

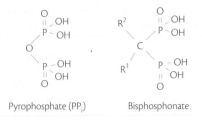

Pyrophosphate (PP$_i$)   Bisphosphonate

Fig. 4.1 Basic bisphosphonate structure compared to pyrophosphate.

bond, which makes them more resistant to breakdown. The structure of a bisphosphonate molecule is shown in Fig. 4.1. The different side-chains to the molecule determine how strongly the bisphosphonate bonds to bone and how potent its effects are.

Bisphosphonates reduce osteoclastic bone breakdown. This increases BMD and decreases bone turnover. Osteoclasts are inhibited when they come into contact with bisphosphonate-containing bone. Bisphosphonates bind into bone and, therefore, retain activity even after the medication is discontinued.

Bisphosphonates can be split into two groups:

◆ the non-nitrogen-containing (Etidronate, Tiludronate and Clodronate); and

◆ the nitrogen-containing compounds (Alendronate, Risedronate, Ibandronate and Zoledronate).

These two groups work in a slightly different way. The nitrogen-containing group has more powerful effects and, therefore, most of the commonly used bisphosphonates are nitrogen-containing.

Bisphosphonates are poorly absorbed, especially in the elderly. They must be given fasted. They bind to bone because of their attraction for calcium and they stay in the skeleton for a long time. They are absorbed, stored, and excreted by the kidney, unaltered by the body. Side-effects are largely those of gastrointestinal upset, especially in the nitrogen-containing bisphosphonate group, which has been known to cause severe heartburn and indigestion. Bisphosphonates are not recommended in pregnancy.

Etidronate

The original bisphosphonate etidronate (Didronal PMO®) is given in a cyclical fashion, for 2 weeks in every 3 months, and increases in spinal BMD of 3–6% over 2 years have been recorded with vertebral fracture rate reductions.

There is no definite evidence of a reduction in hip fractures. Whilst an effective agent in vertebral fracture prevention, it has been largely superseded by the more potent bisphosphonates.

Pamidronate

Pamidronate has been shown to be effective in treating those with vertebral fractures. The main side-effect experienced with it is a transient episode of fever and chills in about 30% of subjects. This intravenous preparation is not licensed in osteoporosis, although it is commonly used in Paget's disease. It has been used 'off licence' in those who fail to tolerate oral bisphosphonates. However, 3-monthly Ibandronate injections (Bonviva®) and annual Zoledronic acid infusions (Aclasta ®) are now available, thus the use of pamidronate in this situation will probably decline.

Alendronate and Risedronate

Alendronate (Fosamax ®; Merck, Sharp & Dohme) and risedronate (Actonel ®; Procter & Gamble) are licensed for use in the prevention and treatment of osteoporosis and in steroid osteoporosis. They reduce the incidence of vertebral and non-vertebral fractures in those with a pre-existing vertebral fracture. Risedronate therapy appears to have its effects within 6 months of onset of therapy and only those who are osteoporotic, as defined by DXA scan, or who have had a previous vertebral fracture show evidence of hip fracture reduction.

Current recommendations for use of these medications are for 10 years continuous therapy with adequate calcium and vitamin D intake. After 10 years of therapy, a treatment-free window of 1–2 years could be considered due to the build up in bone of these medications. To date, 10 years of alendronate therapy has not been shown to be associated with any abnormal bone effects.

Alendronate and risedronate would be considered as comparable medications and are the mainstay of current management in osteoporosis. However, in many countries, including the UK, alendronate is now a generic drug and is produced by many pharmaceutical companies rather than the company that initially arranged the research studies and marketed the drug. The result is that alendronate is often as little as 10% of the cost of the original proprietary brand and most patients will be offered it as the first treatment option. The medications are taken by mouth, once per week, fasted, at least 30 min before the first food of the day. The commonest reported side-effects are of gastrointestinal upset, particularly heartburn or indigestion. Perhaps as many as 1 in 100 people cannot tolerate these medications because of gastrointestinal upset.

Table 4.6 Types of bisphosphonates

Oral	Intravenous
Alendronate	Pamidronate
Risedronate	Zoledronate
Ibandronate	Ibandronate
Etidronate	

Ibandronate and zoledronate

Ibandronate (Bonviva®; Roche) and zoledronate or zoledronic acid (Aclasta®; Novartis), are both nitrogen-containing bisphosphonates. Zoledronate is an intravenous preparation given once yearly by infusion. It has been shown to be effective in preventing vertebral and hip fractures. It is licensed for use in both Paget's disease of bone and in bone cancers, as well as in osteoporosis. There is some evidence that it increases life-expectancy by decreasing cardiovascular episodes in an elderly population.

Ibandronate is available both as a once per month tablet and as a 3-monthly injection. Both oral and intravenous Ibandronate appear to be effective in the prevention of fractures in osteoporosis, although there is as yet no evidence of whether it would be effective in preventing hip fractures. The benefit of a monthly tablet might be improvements in the numbers of individuals taking their tablets regularly. Currently it is recognized that only around 3–4 of every 10 people take their medications on a regular basis. The intravenous medications prevent gut side-effects in those who cannot tolerate oral bisphosphonate tablets.

Intravenous bisphosphonates have no gastrointestinal side-effects. However, they can be associated with what is termed an acute phase response: flu-like reaction in the 24–48 hours following the first infusion/injection, which is far less marked with subsequent injections. Subjects complain of feeling achy

Table 4.7 Side-effects of bisphosphonates

Oral	Intravenous
Gastrointestinal upset	Inflammation of the eye
Inflammation of the eye	Acute phase response
Skin rashes	Osteonecrosis of jaw (rare)

and shivery as though they have a viral infection. Simply co-prescribing paracetamol at the time of the first injection can reduce these side-effects. (Tables 4.6, 4.7).

Rarely, a condition called osteonecrosis of the jaw, in which an ulcer forms on the jaw bone, has been observed in patients receiving high doses of very strong, usually intravenous, bisphosphonates. These occurrences have been most commonly, but not exclusively, seen in bone cancer patients. It is clearly a very rare event in patients receiving treatment for osteoporosis. It is, however, recommended that patients with poor dental hygiene do not receive intravenous bisphosphonates.

📄 Case study

A 64-year-old woman with a known history of osteoporosis presented to her doctor with severe back pain. She has been taking an oral bisphosphonate medication for 2 years and, additionally, was on a calcium and vitamin D supplement. Her own doctor referred her for a spinal X-ray, which revealed the presence of two new vertebral fractures.

In the past she also had a history of pancreatic disease and a history of malabsorption of food.

She had a follow-up DXA scan, which showed signs of deterioration of her bone density, despite taking her medications regularly and as prescribed. It was decided that she might not be absorbing her tablets properly and was, therefore, changed onto an intravenous bisphosphonate instead. Her bone density and biochemical tests improved with this change in medication and she has suffered no further fractures to this day.

Selective oestrogen-receptor antagonists (SERMS)

The anti-oestrogenic drug tamoxifen is widely used to prevent recurrence of some types of breast cancer. While tamoxifen is anti-oestrogenic in breast tissue, it has positive oestrogen effects on bone and, therefore, reduces bone breakdown in a similar manner to HRT. Tamoxifen, however, is oestrogenic to the lining of the womb and hence there is an increased risk of developing endometrial cancer. Tamoxifen, while beneficial to bone in post-menopausal women, is not licensed for the prevention or treatment of osteoporosis.

Raloxifene is a similar agent, a selective oestrogen-receptor modulator (SERM). It binds to oestrogen receptors and reduces bone breakdown with no adverse effects on the lining of the womb in post-menopausal women. Over 7000 women were studied in the major raloxifene studies, which concluded that raloxifene reduced the incidence of new vertebral fractures in those with and without previous vertebral fractures. However, there was no reduction in the incidence of non-vertebral fractures (i.e. hip fractures). No endometrial problems were encountered, although women were more likely to experience hot flushes while taking raloxifene, compared to taking dummy tablets. Leg cramps and mild ankle swelling were also reported and it should be noted that raloxifene increases the risk of venous clotting in the same way as does HRT (Table 4.8). Women with a history of deep venous thrombosis should, therefore, avoid raloxifene. Of particular note, however, in the raloxifene studies was the 90% decrease in breast cancers. Overall the risk of breast cancer was decreased by 76% during 3 years of treatment with raloxifene. Raloxifene has been available in the UK since September 1998.

Other antiresorptive drugs
Calcitonin

Calcitonin continues to have a place in the management of osteoporosis but the role is tertiary to the bisphosphonates, HRT, and SERMS.

Calcitonin is a naturally occurring hormone produced by the thyroid gland. It exerts its calcium-lowering effects by reducing bone breakdown and is currently available as an intramuscular or nasal spray preparation. It is possible that with time antibodies form against the calcitonin, which may diminish its effect.

Calcitonin has been found to reduce bone loss. Nasal calcitonin appears to reduce vertebral fracture risk but there is no convincing evidence of hip fracture prevention. It may be that effects of calcitonin are effects on bone quality, rather than bone quantity. Unique amongst osteoporosis therapies it appears to reduce the pain after an acute vertebral fracture.

Table 4.8 Side-effects of SERMs

Side-effects
Hot flushes
Leg cramps
Ankle swelling
Increased risk of venous blood clotting

Anabolic therapies
Parathyroid hormone analogues

Parathyroid hormone (PTH) is a hormone made by the parathyroid glands, which has complex effects on bone. Continuous PTH secretion results in reduced bone formation, whereas intermittent PTH leads to increased bone formation. PTH stimulates bone resorption by an indirect route, via the osteoblasts, which send signals in turn to the osteoclasts.

The first indication that PTH injections could have an anabolic (bone-forming) effect on bone emerged some 70 years ago. It was soon realized that intermittent, rather than continuous, exposure to PTH was required for its bone-forming effects.

Treatment with PTH has major effects on bone remodelling within 1 month of starting therapy, with maximum effects apparent by 6 months.

Studies in growing rats have revealed an increased incidence in the development of a rare bone cancer called osteosarcoma, which appeared to be related to both the duration of treatment and the dose of PTH used in the study. Therefore, PTH therapy is not suitable for use in children and only licensed for an 18-month course of therapy. There is no evidence of bone cancers in humans.

PTH analogues are licensed in the UK for treatment of severe post-menopausal osteoporosis. Given by daily self-administered subcutaneous (just under the skin) injection for 18 months, the effects on both BMD and fracture reduction have exceeded other bone therapies. The side-effect profile of PTH analogues is excellent, with most patients tolerating these drugs with no side-effects (Table 4.9).

It has been found that patients pre-treated with a bisphosphonate do not show the same degree of improvements in bone thickness with PTH analogues. Raloxifene pre-treatment does not seem to have a negative effect on subsequent PTH therapy. This has led many physicians to recommend a 6-month window, bisphosphonate-free, before commencing a PTH analogue.

Table 4.9 Side-effects of PTH analogues

Injection site reactions
Dizziness/vertigo
Muscle cramps
Depression

After the 18-month course of a PTH analogue, it is recommended that a further antiresorptive therapy, such as a bisphosphonate, be prescribed to maintain the improvements seen after the PTH analogue.

Human PTH therapies are manufactured by genetic engineering and, therefore, are very costly therapies. Although approved for use in the UK, in many areas local funding for therapy has not become available. They are restricted for use in those with severe osteoporosis who cannot tolerate bisphosphonate therapy, or who have experienced low trauma fractures despite bisphosphonate therapy.

Case study

Mrs B, a 68-year-old woman, was diagnosed 3 years previously with severe osteoporosis. She had suffered a previous wrist fracture and had an early menopause at the age of 40. She did not receive treatment with HRT.

At the time of her diagnosis she was started on an oral bisphosphonate and additionally given calcium and vitamin D supplements. She took her medications as prescribed and they did not upset her. Unfortunately, following a simple trip she had a further wrist fracture after 2 years of treatment. Mrs B had a follow-up DXA scan but no improvements were seen in the bone thickness.

Her doctor explained that her medications were not working adequately and asked her to stop her bisphosphonate. A period of 6 months then passed until she was ready to commence a PTH analogue treatment. Mrs B was extremely anxious about this but she was taught to self-inject by nurses who came to her home, and whom she was able to contact whenever she had any concerns. She quickly became very proficient at the self-injection technique. The medication stopped after 18 months of treatment and she was delighted when her follow-up bone scan showed a 14% improvement in the bone mass of her spine.

Mrs B recommenced her oral bisphosphonate once she had completed the PTH injections and in a further 2 years of follow-up has not had any further fractures.

Strontium ranelate

This compound is incorporated into the structure of bone and binds to its surface. The effect is to prevent the osteoclasts from breaking down bone efficiently, and this occurs without impeding the ability of osteoblasts from making new bone. This fact leads to the inclusion of this medication as a new class of drug—a dual-action bone agent (DABA)—as, although it reduces osteoclast activity, it also increases osteoblast activity, at least in animal studies.

Good bone mass improvements have been found with this therapy; however, some of this is artificial, being caused because strontium is a heavy metal with a higher atomic weight than calcium.

Strontium therapy reduces the incidence of vertebral and peripheral fractures and hip fracture incidence. It cannot be monitored by either a DXA scan, due to its artefact on BMD measurements, or by biochemical markers of bone turnover, where the changes are too small to assess. The bone density will, however, increase as recorded with a DXA scan and this will at least indicate that the medication has been absorbed successfully. There is some indication that the increases in bone mass seen with a DXA scan do relate to improvements in fracture rates.

📄 Case study

Ms W is an 85-year-old woman who lives in a residential home and has done so for 3 years. She fell whilst trying to go to the toilet one night and broke her right hip.

Ms W struggles with her health, having additionally a degree of heart failure, and takes numerous medications. She is generally rather frail and prone to falling.

She was even frailer after her discharge from the orthopaedic department after having her hip fracture pinned.

She was not fit enough to attend her local DXA scanning department but her GP felt she should be given some medication to try and prevent further fractures. She experienced quite marked heartburn with an oral bisphosphonate and instead was started on strontium ranelate therapy. She found this lemon-flavoured drink before bedtime was quite pleasant and it did not appear to upset her at all. As she was falling regularly, she was also supplied with hip protector pants and a physiotherapist came to the home to try and improve her safety when walking with her zimmer frame.

Table 4.10 Side-effects of strontium ranelate

Nausea
Diarrhoea
Rashes
Increased venous blood clotting

Strontium must be taken fasted, 2 hours after the last food of the day. Commonest side-effects of this sachet dissolved in water are diarrhoea, nausea, and skin rashes. If a rash occurs when taking this medication, the medication should be discontinued immediately. In some studies it has also been associated with an increased risk of venous blood clotting (Table 4.10).

Strontium ranelate is licensed for use in the UK, but restricted to those who have experienced a fracture, have confirmed osteoporosis, are unable to take a bisphosphonate, and are over the age of 75 years.

Guidelines

Many guidelines for healthcare professionals now exist in the field of osteoporosis. The National Osteoporosis Society has been instrumental in bring about many of these guidelines with position statements on ultrasound and peripheral devices in the investigation of osteoporosis, on paediatric assessments, DXA scanning and reporting, and, in 1998, released guidance on the management of steroid-induced osteoporosis based on the evidence available at that stage. This advocated the use of DXA scanning for those commencing steroids to identify bone mass and to initiate treatment in those at future risks. The intervention level is higher than in patients without steroid therapy, recognising the added risks of steroid medication on future fracture risk. More formalized guidelines were released by the Royal College of Physicians in December 2002 (in collaboration with the NOS and the Bone and Tooth Society of Great Britain).

In Scotland advice stems from SIGN (Scottish Intercollegiate Guidelines Network) and guidelines on osteoporosis (SIGN 71) were published in June 2003, and hip fracture guidelines (No. 56) were issued in January 2002, replacing the original guideline (No. 15). The Scottish Medicines consortium has also produced guidance on the use of bisphosphonates, teriparatide, and strontium ranelate therapy.

In the UK, the decision as to which drug to use in which circumstances is governed by the National Institute of Health and Clinical Excellence (NICE). NICE reported on secondary fracture prevention in January 2005 as a Health Technology Assessment (HTA) guidance, which needs to be implemented across the UK. A NICE clinical guideline is advisory but it is not mandatory for the advice to be implemented. NICE Guideline 21 gives advice on the assessment and treatment of falls in older people. NICE have also produced a draft HTA guidance for primary fracture prevention advice (for those with osteoporosis who have not as yet experienced a fracture) and an updated secondary prevention HTA guidance, but these are still under discussion. Much controversy was raised by these initial NICE drafts, which suggested alendronate as the mainstay of management of osteoporosis, based on cost issues. Whilst alendronate is an effective agent in osteoporosis, not all patients can tolerate it and other therapies need to be available in those who cannot.

The Department of Health document *National Service framework for older people* serves to look at the problems experienced by older people and to eradicate age discrimination and support person-centred integrated services. Falls prevention is considered within the service framework.

New treatments for the future?

There is much active research in the field of bone health and many exciting opportunities for the development of new medications for osteoporosis. Much of this research is focused on the new understandings of the mechanisms leading to bone thinning, allowing targeting of new therapies. Some of these exciting areas are discussed below but it must be remembered that not all exciting research ideas come to fruition and eventually lead to new therapeutic approaches (Table 4.11).

Table 4.11 New therapeutic areas in osteoporosis

Novel vitamin D analogues
Regulators of bone turnover: denosumab
Selective oestrogen receptor modulators
Selective androgen-receptor modulators
Cathepsin K inhibitors: balicatib
Wnt signalling pathway

Novel vitamin D analogues

The effects of vitamin D on bone and calcium metabolism are via a receptor found on many cells. New molecules that resemble vitamin D have been found, which bind very effectively to the vitamin D receptor and have enhanced effects compared to naturally occurring vitamin D, without apparently causing the main expected side-effect of too high blood calcium levels. One such molecule has been found that can increase the bone density in rats by some 10%. This area of research is at a preliminary stage but is of great interest.

Newly identified regulators of bone turnover

One of the major advances in bone biology in the last decade has been the identification of receptor activator of nuclear factor kappa B (RANK) and its ligand (RANKL) as key regulators of bone turnover. RANKL is a factor secreted by osteoblasts (bone-forming cells) in response to numerous signals and this factor regulates the activity of osteoclasts (bone breakdown cells). RANKL binds to a receptor on the osteoclast called RANK. Another 'dummy' receptor exists called osteoprotegerin (OPG), which can block the effects of RANKL. Anything that blocks RANKL will lead to less bone breakdown.

Compounds have been developed that do block RANKL or inhibit it. One such preparation termed Denosumab and made by the Amgen Corp is being studied in human subjects with bone thinning now. This is a fully humanized monoclonal synthetic antibody (i.e. one that is nearly identical to what might occur naturally in humans), which binds to RANKL with high affinity and specificity, and blocks the activation of RANK. The medication is given by injection once every 6 months. The effects on bone density and bone turnover appear, at this stage, to be comparable (or a little greater), to those of an oral bisphosphonate, and the side-effects of the medication seem similar in the active and placebo arms of the study. Much larger and longer studies are now underway to determine how useful such a medication will be and whether the positive biochemical changes translate into reduced risk of fractures in study subjects.

This area of study seems very promising for further therapies.

Selective oestrogen-receptor modulators and selective androgen-receptor modulators

The currently available SERM (raloxifene) does have positive bone effects but induces menopausal symptoms and increases blood-clotting risks. New SERMS are under development. Currently three are undergoing final-stage human studies. Several other SERMS have been studied but have not been successful, usually because of adverse effects on the lining of the womb. It is know that the 'original' SERM, tamoxifen, can cause problems to the lining of the womb. Preliminary data with one of the newly developed compounds (lasofoxifene) suggests it is superior to raloxifene in changing bone markers and increasing bone density.

Selective androgen-receptor modulators (SARMS) have been studied for some time, initially in the area of male contraception and treatment of prostate cancers. A current product under study appears to have a positive effect of bone without any negative effects on male sexual function or prostatic cancer incidence.

There is evidence from animal studies that SERMS and SARMS might have positive effects on bone in both sexes, but much more work is required in this area before the drugs become available for clinical use.

Wnt signalling pathways

These are pathways in bone involved in the regulation of osteoblasts (bone-forming cells). They are important in determining bone strength and mass. A genetic study of a family with high bone mass reported in 1997, found a high bone mass gene on chromosome 11. Further refining of the genetic analysis identified a gene (the *LRP5* gene) and this gene is a member of the Wnt signalling pathway. The proteins involved in this pathway have been identified. It is known that these proteins regulate OPG (the secreted protein that inhibits bone resorption), as well as increasing bone formation. Many companies have been looking for compounds that will influence Wnt signalling pathways to treat osteoporosis. Currently an antibody against sclerostin, one of the Wnt signalling proteins, has been giving encouraging results in mice studies. Human medications are still some way off, however.

Cathepsin K inhibitors

Cathepsin K is an enzyme produced by osteoclasts that assists in bone breakdown. It particularly breaks down type 1 collagen. Cathepsin K inhibitors reduce bone resorption but not bone formation. Balicatib, an investigational cathepsin K inhibitor, has been shown to reduce bone resorption but not bone formation, with good bone mineral density increases seen. Much work is being done in this area and phase 2 human studies are underway. Phase 2 studies are those in which the best dose of drug for a combination of efficacy and safety is tested, while phase 3 are the trials that are planned to persuade regulatory authorities to give a licence to the product provided the trial is successful.

➲ Summary

- Bone metabolism is an area where rapid research findings based on basic scientific studies are being translated into possible new therapeutic strategies for patients with bone diseases such as osteoporosis, Paget's disease, and bone cancers.

- Bisphosphonates will provide the main therapeutic options for therapy in the coming years either with oral or intravenous preparations but the future seems bright for other approaches for the management of bone.

5

Diet, exercise, smoking, alcohol, and prevention of falls

⤵ Key points

- A balanced diet rich in calcium is recommended for healthy bones.

- Vitamin D is important for bone health.

- People who have healthy bones and are eating a healthy diet, do not need to take supplements.

- People with osteoporosis are usually prescribed calcium and vitamin D supplements.

- Exercise is important for bone health, as well as general health.

- Weight-bearing exercise stimulates bone density to prevent thin bones.

- Different levels of exercise are beneficial, depending on age group.

- Smoking affects bone health and support is available to stop smoking.

- Taking too much alcohol is bad for bones and increases the risk of falling.

- The risk of falling increases as we get older but some falls can be prevented.

- Avoid falls by keeping fit, have regular sight tests, keep feet in good condition, and ensure safety in the home.

This chapter will deal with general lifestyle factors that can improve our bone health and also look at mechanisms to reduce the incidence of falls

Most of us feel we would like to do all we can do for ourselves to keep healthy generally and with our bones this is no exception. Lifestyle advice for bone health is also advice for healthy living. Research regarding the impact of lifestyle factors on bone health is sometimes inconclusive but many studies do show that nutrition, exercise, not smoking, and having no more than a moderate intake of alcohol does have a positive impact on bone health.

Although peak bone mass is mainly determined by genetic factors, factors such as good nutrition and taking plenty of exercise influence bone mass in a positive way during this phase of skeletal growth. Lifestyle changes can be very difficult but having healthier and stronger bones makes it worthwhile.

Diet

Good nutrition is a basic requirement for our bodies to function to their optimum levels. Prevention of bone loss through diet is complex and involves many nutrients. Health professionals recommend a balanced diet rich in calcium for bone health.

Calcium

Most of the calcium in our bodies is found in the bones. By having a balanced diet containing all the five food groups (Table 5.1 and Fig. 5.1), other aspects of health will benefit as well as bones. Calcium is important for bones but it is not the only nutrient needed for bone health. Many other nutrients have a part to play and it is likely that they interact together for optimal bone health.

Calcium is essential to give bone the ability to support the body and its weight. Calcium is a component involved in other body functions. It is involved in the correct functioning of the blood and nerve conduction and if any problems

Table 5.1 Food groups

Carbohydrates: bread, potatoes, pasta and cereals.
Fruit and vegetables.
Protein: meat, fish, eggs, pulses, nuts and seeds.
Milk and dairy products.
Fat and sugar.

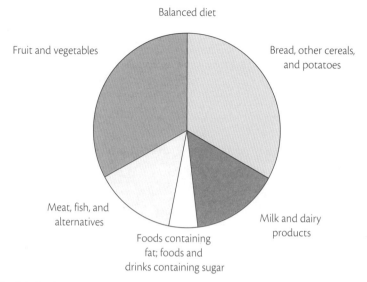

Fig. 5.1 Food groups.

arise with these functions, calcium reserves in the skeleton can be used to prevent life-threatening problems.

The best source of calcium is found in dairy products. Skimmed and semi-skimmed milk, low-fat yoghurt, and low-fat cheese contain as much calcium as full-fat dairy products. Calcium is found in many foods other than dairy products but dairy products contain a higher amount of calcium (Table 5.2).

Other foods containing calcium include:

- In the fruit and vegetable food group: green leafy vegetables, broccoli, spring greens, watercress, curly kale, oranges, apricots, and figs.

- In the protein food group: red kidney beans, green beans, baked beans, fish such as sardines and mackerel, nuts such as brazil nuts and almonds.

- In the carbohydrate food group: breakfast cereals and bread.

Vegetarians or people who avoid taking dairy products because of allergies or dislike of these products can still have a diet containing the recommended intake of calcium with a bit of thought about diet. Tofu is a good source of calcium and many soya-based products have added calcium.

Table 5.2 Calcium Intake

Recommended daily calcium intakes
Adult men and women: 700 mg
Teenage boys: 11–18 years 1000 mg; girls 11–18 years 800 mg
Children 1–3 years: 350 mg
Children 4–6 years: 450 mg
Children 7–10 years: 550 mg
Infants (breast fed only) 0–12 months: 525 mg
Pregnant women: 700 mg

Vitamin D

Vitamin D is a fat-soluble vitamin involved in the absorption of calcium from the intestines. Most of our vitamin D is obtained from the action of sunlight on the skin. The ultraviolet rays from the sun result in the inactive form of vitamin D, cholecalciferol, being formed in the skin. It is then absorbed into the bloodstream, the muscles, and fat and passes through the liver and kidneys to become the active form of vitamin D (1,25-dihydroxyvitamin D), which is used in the body. It is not possible for too much vitamin D to be formed in this way. It is recommended that in the United Kingdom we should expose our face, legs, and arms to the sun during the summer months for about 15 min before applying sunscreen.

Vitamin D is also found in some foods such as egg yolks, oily fish such as herrings and mackerel, and it is usually added to margarine. Only 10% of our intake of vitamin D comes from nutrition, the rest is obtained from sunlight.

The recommended daily dose in the United Kingdom for vitamin D intake is 10 μg or 400 IU. It may be that in the future this recommendation will change, as some nutritionists think that this daily intake should be higher.

Vitamin D can help to improve muscles and balance. It is thought that having an adequate intake of vitamin D can help to reduce the risk of falling in older people.

Lack of vitamin D can lead to less calcium being available for the bones leading to osteomalacia in adults and rickets in children. Too much vitamin D, from tablet supplements, causes hypercalcaemia (too much calcium in the blood).

People at risk of not getting enough vitamin D are those who are housebound or wear dress where they are covered up and skin is not exposed. Also people who have heavy skin pigmentation in this country would need longer in the sun because melanin in the skin competes for the UV rays of the sun.

Supplements of calcium and vitamin D

The most efficient way to obtain calcium and vitamin D is by eating a healthy diet and being active outdoors. However, for people with an inadequate dietary intake or with osteoporosis, calcium and vitamin D supplementation may be necessary. For adults with osteoporosis it is usual to prescribe 500–1000 mg of calcium and 400–800 IU of vitamin D daily; this may vary depending on the amount of calcium taken in the diet. Calcium supplements should not be taken at the same time of day as iron supplements, bisphosphonates, or strontium ranelate.

It is recommended not to have more than 2000 mg of calcium daily, including diet. It may be that much higher amounts will increase the risk of developing kidney stones. Having a high calcium intake does not prevent osteoporosis— genetic factors have a stronger influence.

Exercise

How does exercise affect bones?

When bones are subjected to forces causing mechanical stress and strain on the bone, the pull of muscles and gravity, bone cells are stimulated and respond by increasing bone density and in turn increasing the strength of the bones. This also means that if the bones are not stimulated in this way, bone density decreases. Bone quality and structure also determine bone strength. Bone structure varies according to the type of bone, where it is in the skeleton, and the stress put on it. So taking part in weight-bearing exercise is important to stimulate bone density and strength, thereby preventing thinning of the bones and maintaining bone density for those who have osteoporosis. The mechanism by which this process works has been demonstrated in research with athletes, where bone density has been shown to be thicker in the serving arm of a tennis player because of the stresses and strains taken by the arm. In contrast, astronauts who have experienced weightlessness in space have been shown to lose bone density during prolonged weightlessness.

Bones are stimulated to grow stronger when they are subjected to any force, which puts strain on bone and resistance to the pull of gravity. Exercise needs to be tailored to suit the needs of the individual. It is always best to check with your doctor before starting any new exercise programmes.

Weight-bearing exercise

The benefits gained by exercising to maintain bone density have to be sustained, otherwise the benefit is lost.

Tai Chi has been shown in research studies to reduce the risk of falling by improving balance. However, for Tai Chi to be of benefit, a certain level of balance fitness is required to do the exercises. One-to-one supervision would be required for someone with poor balance.

Young adults

Exercise in young adults is especially significant because bones are in the process of developing and achieving peak bone density. Young people can take part in exercises that are more high impact, such as jogging, aerobics, and athletics.

Osteoporosis

Exercise for people with osteoporosis should be tailored to avoid harm or injury. People with osteoporosis should avoid the following movements:

- any movement involving twisting of the spine;

- bending forward from the waist with straight legs;

- sit-ups;

- touching the toes;

- lifting heavy weights.

The National Osteoporosis Society has published a booklet for exercise and osteoporosis.

Smoking

Smoking tobacco remains the single greatest cause of preventable ill health and early death in the United Kingdom. Smoking has a role to play in cancer, chest disease, heart disease, and strokes. In the case of osteoporosis, smoking affects bones at a cellular level by reducing the action of the osteoblasts, the cells that build new bone. By stopping smoking, bone density will benefit, as well as other aspects of general health.

Most health authorities have Smoking Advice Services to provide information and support for those who wish to stop smoking. Smoking cessation advisors will assess the needs of the individual and provide the support required. This can range from simple discussion to fully supported structured programmes of smoking cessation. Individuals are all different and some will need more support than others. Advice services also give information on nicotine replacement therapy. This comes in the form of patches, gum, inhalers, microtabs, lozenges, and nasal sprays. Pharmacists in the community can also give information and advice on nicotine replacement therapy.

Alcohol

It is a fact that in the United Kingdom people are drinking more alcohol more frequently. There is a growing culture of binge-drinking, especially among younger people. Excessive alcohol use affects the skin, liver, stomach, pancreas, brain, nervous system, heart and circulatory system, and the reproductive system.

For bones, taking too much alcohol increases the risk of falling and breaking bones. People who take too much alcohol often do not eat properly. This can lead to problems with nutrition affecting bones in a negative way, when the nutrients required for bone health are not available. However, in moderation alcohol consumption can be compatible with a healthy lifestyle.

It is important to know the strength of the alcohol by volume (%abv). It is no longer accurate to say one glass of wine is equal to one unit. The system for measuring drinks was introduced over 20 years ago and there have been developments in strength and variety of alcohol products.

Prevention of falls

Falls can happen for many reasons. In fact, children and athletes fall more than elderly people but the difference is that the effect of falling is much more serious for an elderly person due to injury. The risk of having a fall increases

Table 5.3 Suggested limits to alcohol intake

Women: 2–3 units per day but not every day and no more than 14 units in total per week.
Men: 3–4 units per day but not every day and no more than 21 units total per week.

the older one becomes. There are many risks for having a fall but age is one of the strongest risks. Falls are a major cause of fractures in people who have osteoporosis. Falls are not random events and are not just 'something that happens' in old age. Women are more at risk of falling than men because their patterns of activity usually differ. Healthy women living in the community are at less risk of having a fall than a woman who is frail and housebound or living in a nursing home. A fall can often be a sign that there is something physically wrong and your GP should be informed, as he may want to investigate this further. It is known that taking four or more medications can increase risk. Some medications have side-effects that cause dizziness making a person more likely to fall. If you let your doctor know if you experience any side-effects with your medication, he will usually be able to prescribe an alternative or reduce the current dose. Falls can happen in the home or outside and in any weather. If you have had a fall and are concerned you should speak to your doctor and nurse.

What can my doctor do to prevent falls?

If you have had a fall, your doctor will ask you for details of what happened. Your doctor will want to know the following about any falls you have had:

◆ Do you remember feeling any physical symptoms before having a fall, for example, were you feeling dizzy?

◆ How many falls have you had in the previous year?

◆ Where did your falls happen, for example, at home or out of doors?

◆ What were you doing at the time?

◆ What time of day did the fall happen?

◆ Were you injured?

Your doctor may want to check your blood pressure and further tests may be recommended depending on any symptoms you may have had before the fall.

Your doctor may ask if you would like a home safety assessment carried out by an occupational therapist. It may be recommended that you attend for an assessment by a physiotherapist. A physiotherapist will decide if you will benefit from exercises and training to improve your balance and strengthen your muscles in order to reduce the risk of falling.

Ways you can help to prevent falls

Nobody likes to think that they may fall but there are steps that can be taken to prevent the likelihood of falls.

- Keeping fit by walking, gardening, swimming, and other activities improves muscle strength and helps to improve balance. Some balance problems can be helped with exercise and instruction from a physiotherapist.

- Vision plays a part in keeping upright and maintaining balance. Annual eye-checks are free to the over-60s. It is advisable not to wear reading glasses, bifocals, or varifocals out of doors. This type of visual aid tends to affect distance and make things seem closer than they actually are. For example, it would be easy to stumble if the edge of a step or stair appeared closer than in reality.

- At home there are common sense precautions that can be taken to avoid falls. Having well-lit areas, such as the stairs, and having a clutter-free home can make a difference to the risk of falling. An occupational therapist can advise on safety in the home.

- Healthy feet are important, as painful feet and conditions like corns and bunions can affect stability. Ill-fitting shoes and slippers have been shown to contribute to risk of falling.

- Fear of falling can be an issue for many people. Some people who have never had a fall worry about this, as do those who have already had a fall. The result is a loss of confidence, causing a restriction in activity. If this happens it should be discussed with a health professional who can give advice on how to increase confidence.

- The charity Help the Aged have produced some excellent information on avoiding falls and safety in the home.

Summary

- There are many things we can do in our own lives to improve our bone health.

- Taking regular weight-bearing exercise, reducing our risk of falling in the home, not drinking to excess, and having a good calcium intake in our diet will all have a positive benefit in preventing future osteoporotic fractures.

6

Osteoporotic fractures

➡ Key points

- ◆ An older person is more at risk of having a fracture if they had a parent who has had a fracture or if the person has osteoporosis and is prone to having falls.

- ◆ Wrist, hip, and spine fractures are the most common fractures.

- ◆ Back pain is a common condition that is often unexplained.

- ◆ Back pain due to spinal fractures may be short-lived or never resolve.

- ◆ Pain can be managed to improve quality of life.

- ◆ Medications to relieve pain should be taken as prescribed.

- ◆ Different types of medication can be used according to the intensity and duration of the pain.

- ◆ There are other effective ways of dealing with pain, as well as taking medication.

- ◆ Coping with chronic pain may mean adapting some aspects of daily living to have the best quality of life possible.

In this chapter we will discuss the types of fractures that occur with osteoporosis and the reasons behind them. Additionally we will look at the treatments available for such fractures.

Fractures

One in two women and one in five men over the age of 50 are at risk of a fracture (broken bone) due to osteoporosis. This is a greater risk for women than having breast cancer or cardiovascular disease. Fractures are the main consequence of osteoporosis. The lower the bone density, the greater the risk of fracture, but fracture does not depend entirely on having a low bone density. Genetic predisposition, older age, and how likely we are to fall are the main risks for having an osteoporotic fracture.

◆ Genetics. Research studies with families and twins have shown that osteoporosis and the risk of having a fracture has a large genetic component. Genetic research has concluded that there is no single identifiable gene that is associated with osteoporosis; there are many genes contributing to the condition. It is known that a person's risk of hip fracture is increased if a parent has had a hip fracture after the age of 50, but there is no one genetic test for osteoporosis.

◆ Age. This factor is actually more important than measurement of bone density when predicting risk of fracture. The older an individual, the thinner bones become, and the risk of fracture increases as we age. It is a natural part of ageing that we lose about 0.5–1% bone density every year from middle age onwards, with slightly more rapid change after the menopause in women. Any deterioration in general health as we age, such as conditions affecting mobility or multiple medications, adds to the risk. Lack of exercise and reduced mobility leads to further bone loss.

◆ Falling. Any condition affecting the ability to mobilize safely, such as Parkinson's Disease or Arthritis, increases the risk of falling. Some medications can make an individual feel dizzy and therefore more prone to falling. Environmental factors both inside and outside the home can increase risk. Falling is very common after the age of 65, one-third of this age group fall every year although not all suffer injury. Prevention of falls is discussed in Chapter 5.

It is possible that someone with all the above risk factors will never have a fracture, equally it is possible that a fracture can occur in those with no risk factors.

Fractures due to osteoporosis occur as a result of reduced bone strength, where a bone is subjected to a force greater than that which it can resist. In other words, a bone can break as the result of a simple fall such as slipping on ice. A fracture is confirmed by having an X-ray. Spinal fractures can also be identified on lateral bone density scans. Osteoporotic fractures can affect any bone in the body but the most common sites are the wrist, hip, and spine. Prevention of fractures is important because the risk of having another fracture increases two to five times more after having the first fracture. However, it should be remembered that risk factors do not cause fractures but just make fractures more likely to happen.

Wrist fractures

Wrist fractures related to osteoporosis more commonly occur in women aged between 40 and 65, and in men over 60, although they can occur at any age. Men are usually genetically predisposed to have bigger and stronger wrists than women and this is why wrist fractures occur later in life for men. Wrist fractures usually occur due to a fall outdoors, such as a fall in winter on an icy pavement. They are usually caused by a fall onto the outstretched hand to save oneself and, therefore, are less common in the elderly.

In some cases, the fracture may need a surgical operation requiring admission to an orthopaedic ward but usually it is treated on an outpatient basis in the Accident and Emergency Department. A plaster cast is applied to the wrist for 4–6 weeks and the patient attends the department several times in the following weeks.

Hip fractures

These happen more frequently in the over-75 age group. In the UK, hip fracture patients occupy 1 in every 5 beds in orthopaedic wards. Most hip fractures are usually caused by a fall within the home.

A hip fracture will require a surgical operation to stabilize the fracture. Depending on the type of fracture sustained, the operation may involve either having metal screws, with or without a metal plate, inserted in the hip; or replacement with an artificial joint. It is usual to start mobilizing soon after surgery in order to avoid any complications and start rehabilitation. Unfortunately, research has shown that following hip fracture, half of all individuals are left with some disability affecting their daily activities. To reduce the chance of any disability, physiotherapists are very involved after surgery in helping to encourage walking, strengthen muscles, and promote recovery. Assistance in walking is required in the initial stages of rehabilitation and the hip fracture patient will be helped to progress from using a walking frame to walking sticks, and then to independent mobility. It may take some weeks or months of rehabilitation to regain full mobility. Some hip fracture patients may not fully regain the mobility they enjoyed before their fracture. This may lead to a need for additional help within the community services.

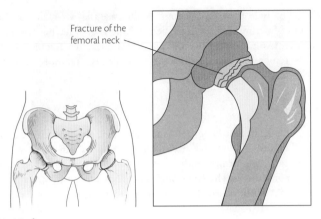

Fig. 6.1 Hip fracture.

Spinal (vertebral) fractures

Research has shown that spinal fractures often occur while performing routine everyday activities, such as lifting a light load, rather than having a fall, as happens mostly with hip and wrist fractures. When a bone in the spine fractures, the bone will collapse and change shape. Kyphosis or Dowager's hump refers to curvature of the spine. Spinal fractures can cause loss of height and kyphosis because it is not possible for the spinal bone to return to the shape it was before the fracture. It is thought that in about half of all spinal fractures there are no symptoms, such as pain or deformity. Due to the change in shape of the spinal bones, the back muscles have to work harder and this can lead to chronic pain. X–rays are the best form of diagnosis for spinal fractures but fractures can also be identified by lateral bone density scanning. Treatment of spinal fractures is focused on pain control and rehabilitation. There are surgical treatments for vertebral fractures that can be carried out by specialist orthopaedic surgeons and radiologists, in some circumstances, but they are not required for the majority of subjects suffering from a fracture.

Treatment of fracture

The aim is initially to stabilize the damage and pain caused by the fracture, either by rest or by surgical intervention, and then medications are used to prevent further bone loss and reduce the risk of future fracture.

◆ Percutaneous vertebroplasty. This is a surgical procedure where the vertebra is repaired by inserting a needle through the skin under the guidance

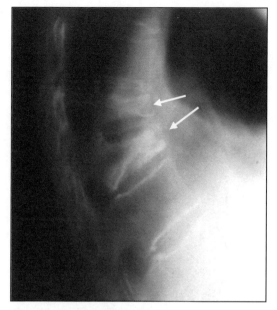

Fig. 6.2 Fracture of the vertebra (spine).

of X-ray and surgical cement is injected into the vertebra to stabilize it. This procedure is most effective when performed within a few weeks of the fracture happening. This procedure may not be suitable if the bone is too fragile.

◆ Percutaneous kyphoplasty. This is a procedure where a small balloon is inserted into the vertebra and it is inflated to try to correct the deformity before the surgical cement is injected.

Both these treatments, as with all surgical procedures, can have complications and risks involved.

The aim of osteoporosis treatment following fracture is to prevent further bone loss and reduce the risk of having another fracture. Osteoporosis treatments are discussed in Chapter 4.

Fracture liaison services

These services are in place in most areas in the UK and usually involve several hospital departments. This model of care identifies men and women over a certain age, usually 55 or 60, who attend hospital after having sustained a low-trauma fracture. Low trauma refers to when a bone is broken when little force has been applied, such as from tripping and falling in the street. These patients are offered osteoporosis assessment, a bone density scan, and education on bone health and the prevention of fractures. Advice and interventions to prevent falls is also a part of many fracture liaison services.

Not everyone who falls and breaks a bone will have osteoporosis and hence the aim of a fracture liaison service is to reduce the risk of future fractures by identifying those who are most at risk, i.e. someone who has already had a fracture and who has osteoporosis. Those who are identified as having osteoporosis can then be treated appropriately to reduce their risk.

At present, the World Health Organization is developing an algorithm to assess a person's risk of having a fracture. This can be used by clinicians to advise people of their chances of having a fracture in the future.

Back pain

What is pain?

The late Patrick Wall, who was an expert in pain management, defined pain as:

> ... an unpleasant sensory or emotional experience associated with actual or potential tissue damage or described in terms of such damage.

What this definition really says is that only the person experiencing pain can describe it.

Back pain is a common condition where only 2% of cases have clear medical disorders, while for others the cause of the back pain is unknown. Changes in the spine due to ageing can cause some back pain. Kyphosis can occur in elderly women without having vertebral deformity and pain is not associated with this unless there is a reduction of height in the vertebral bodies.

How physically fit a person is can have an impact on back pain. Weak muscles in the back and abdomen may not fully support the spine. Other factors affecting back pain include being generally inactive or engaging in sudden or irregular bouts of activity, putting additional strain on the back muscles. Heavy lifting, being overweight, or having a medical condition affecting the bones and muscles, such as arthritis, all put additional strain on back muscles. Stress has an impact on back pain, it can affect the severity of the pain experienced and put pressure on surrounding muscles by making them even more tense and painful.

To reduce or prevent back pain it is important to maintain strong back muscles, this also helps to reduce the risk of falling and fracturing for people with osteoporosis. Exercises like Tai Chi are good for muscle tone, balance, and maintaining a good posture, as is any weight-bearing exercise. More information on exercise is given in Chapter 5. If overweight, losing weight will help take the strain off the spine and other muscles and joints.

Back pain due to spinal fractures

Osteoporosis is a painless condition but pain can arise due to spinal fractures and the associated effects on the surrounding muscles and tissues. Sudden acute back pain can indicate that a spinal fracture has occurred. In someone who has osteoporosis, this can happen spontaneously or as the result of an awkward movement, such as reaching to a high shelf or lifting something heavy. Osteoporotic spinal fractures occur most commonly at the lower part of the spine behind the chest and the upper part of the lumbar spine. Only half of all osteoporosis sufferers complain of back pain after a spinal fracture. The pain felt does not necessarily relate to the number of fractures sustained. Some people may suffer intense pain that can be felt up and down the back and through to the chest with a fracture in one vertebra, whilst others may have several fractures with only mild discomfort. Healing of a spinal fracture should take place within 6 to 12 weeks of the fracture occurring, and any pain should lessen within that time. Some people, however, experience pain for longer or develop chronic pain.

Acute back pain

Acute pain refers to intense pain coming on quickly and may last from a few days to a few weeks. The pain may be constant or intermittent. This type of back pain can be treated with medications and usually resolves when the injury or condition causing the pain is treated. In the case of vertebral fractures, acute pain may last for about 6 weeks and resolve within 3 months. Normal activities may be limited during this time but, as the pain eases, they should be gradually built up again. Bed rest is not recommended, except for as few days as possible after spinal fracture, as directed by a physician. It is best to keep moving gently during this period of healing but it is acceptable to have a couple of rests for twenty minutes or so during the day by lying on top of a bed. This rest period will relax your back and give a renewed bout of energy for the rest of the day.

Chronic back pain

Chronic pain refers to pain continuing after treatment of a condition or healing of an injury is assumed to have occurred. This type of pain may last for months, years or may never resolve. Chronic back pain due to spinal fractures may need other treatments, as well as medications, to help the sufferer cope.

Treatment

Treatment of back pain is most important and it is essential to seek help and learn to manage pain. It may well be that the problem causing the pain cannot be cured, so treating the pain itself is the only option to regain control of one's life. If a person experiences pain over a long time, it may change their normal pattern of life so that they are no longer able to do the things they would normally do in their everyday lives, such as working or socializing with family. This has a knock-on effect in that it only worsens the situation. They may, as a consequence, suffer depression and have difficulty sleeping. This in turn reduces the ability to function properly on a day-to-day basis. Pain from spinal fractures may be further complicated by other conditions such as arthritis of the spine, or other health problems may exacerbate the problem.

Treating back pain should enable improved physical and social function, so that the individual can resume activities within the home and with family. By relieving back pain, sleeping patterns should improve and this promotes higher tolerance of activity during the day. Having adequate sleep means having an increased ability to cope with any residual pain. Ability to function generally improves so that if, for example, a fear of falling has developed, the ability to cope improves. All these factors enhance an individual's quality of life.

Treatment may include taking painkillers to relieve pain, exercise, physiotherapy, and other treatments.

❌ Myths about painkillers

❌ Myth

Many people get addicted to painkillers.

❶ Fact

This is a common misconception because people believe that, because a person may experience withdrawal symptoms when stopping a drug such as an opioid, this constitutes addiction. This physical dependence is a normal response to long-term therapy and symptoms can be reduced if

---

the drug is gradually, not suddenly, stopped. Addiction is defined as continuing to use a drug despite harm to the user or others. For someone experiencing pain, the risk of becoming addicted to pain-killing medications is very small but is obviously higher in someone who has a history of drug abuse.

❌ Myth

Painkillers should only be taken when needed.

❗ Fact

Many people understandably do not want to take any medications unless they feel they really need them but it is well known by health professionals that pain is much more difficult to control if nothing is done about it until it becomes unbearable.

❌ Myth

It is better to just put up with the pain because painkillers may mask a problem or cause more damage.

❗ Fact

It may be thought that pain should just be endured but the fact is that enduring pain only leads to putting more stress on the body, preventing healing, and reducing quality of life. People who have chronic pain should take medication regularly as prescribed so that pain is controlled and they can get on with their lives.

❌ Myth

The side-effects of painkillers are worse than the pain.

❗ Fact

All medications have potential side-effects but it does not follow that every individual will experience those side-effects. However, some people do experience side-effects and this can put them off taking any medication to control pain. Nevertheless it is a fact that there are a lot of medications to choose from when prescribing pain relief, and if a particular medication works well but causes side-effects, there is always the option to continue but, in addition, treat the side-effect as well.

Medications to relieve pain

There is no shame in taking painkillers when recovering from a spinal fracture or when suffering chronic pain. To control pain it is important to take painkillers regularly as prescribed and to strictly follow instructions on how many tablets to take and when to take them.

◆ Sustained-release preparations may be preferable for someone who does not like to take tablets frequently, as these preparations are only taken either once or twice a day.

◆ Consider medications available in liquid form, dispersible, or as patches, if swallowing tablets is difficult.

◆ Simple painkillers such as paracetamol (acetaminophen) or combination painkillers such as co-dydramol, co-codamol, and dihydrocodeine. Preparations containing codeine can cause constipation, so it is also advisable to remember to drink plenty of fluids and to increase dietary fibre. Increasing mobility, once the painkiller is effective, will help to prevent constipation but, if all else fails, it may be useful to ask your doctor about the use of laxatives.

◆ Non-steroidal anti-inflammatory drugs help to control inflammation as well as pain. They include aspirin, ibuprofen, naproxen, and diclofenac. Side-effects include indigestion and so these medications would not be suitable if a person had a history of gastric problems, asthma, or heart disease. Anti-inflammatory drugs may also be prescribed topically.

◆ Stronger painkillers include morphine, fentanyl, and tramadol. These are usually used for a short time when pain is acute; for example, in the first weeks following a spinal fracture. Side-effects, such as nausea and drowsiness, can be treated. The dose of the painkiller can be adjusted and anti-emetics (preventing sickness) can be prescribed.

◆ Anti-depressants, such as amitriptyline, are effective for relieving nerve pain and are usually prescribed in a low dose to start with. They are usually prescribed at night and also to help with sleeping problems. It may be thought that an anti-depressant is only given to improve the mood of the back pain sufferer who may be reluctant to take it, but for pain, these drugs are usually given in smaller doses than would be required as an anti-depressant.

◆ Anti-epileptic drugs such as gabapentin may also be useful for nerve pain.

Other methods for relieving pain

Physiotherapy and exercise

These can help to regain mobility. The physiotherapist can teach exercises to do at home, so that muscles can be strengthened and pain in turn can be reduced. The benefits of exercise are many and include improved balance, co-ordination, and posture. Exercise also helps to prevent health complications incurred by lack of mobility; it also improves self-esteem. Although doing exercises may be difficult when in pain, muscles that are not used can make the pain and disability worse.

Hydrotherapy

Exercising in warm water can be helpful in the early weeks following a spinal fracture. It works because the water causes the body to feel weightless in the water, thereby relieving the stress on muscles and joints. Hydrotherapy can ease aching joints and relax tense muscles, giving confidence to further mobilize after having fractures. Hydrotherapy may not be available in all areas and referral for this treatment needs to come from a GP, physiotherapist, or hospital doctor.

Hot packs

These can be effective in helping with pain. Heat dilates the blood vessels and helps to reduce muscle spasms in the back. Hot packs can usually be heated for a few seconds in the microwave to a temperature preferable to the individual. Instructions for heating a pack should be carefully followed. A hot-water bottle can also be used as a hot pack; both the hot-water bottle and the hot pack should be covered with a towel before use. Care should be taken to prevent damage or burning of the skin. Skin should be clean and dry without oils or creams, which could increase skin sensitivity. A hot pack can be applied to the painful area for 20–30 minutes. Hot packs or hot-water bottles should not be used if there are skin or circulation problems.

Cold packs

Cold packs can help if there is inflammation as well as pain. Cold decreases the blood vessels and numbs the pain. Cold packs should only be used for about 10 minutes at a time and always applied with a cover because applying directly to the skin may cause damage. Cold packs should be examined before use to check for damage or leaks. Again, if there are any skin or circulatory problems, cold pack should never be used.

Transcutaneous electrical nerve stimulation (TENS) machines

These are battery operated and can be worn attached to clothing. Electrodes are placed on the painful areas and the machine has different settings that can be adjusted to suit the individual. Positioning of the electrodes is very much individual choice for effectiveness and the patient may have to experiment with placement to have maximum effect. The machines are thought to work by interfering with the messages sent from nerves to the brain giving the sensation of pain. TENS machines will not cure the pain, they alter the sensation of the pain by producing a tingling feeling instead. TENS machines can be purchased by the individual or obtained on loan from physiotherapists and other hospital departments. People who have pacemakers should not use a TENS machine because it could interfere with the pacemaker due to the electrical impulse produced. The leads of a TENS machine should never be placed over the neck area or on damaged skin. Anyone who suffers from epilepsy should use these machines with care; there may be an additional safety issue if wearing a TENS whilst having a seizure.

Pain clinics

Specialists who are experienced in treating pain run pain clinics in most large hospitals. When a GP or osteoporosis specialist is unable to effectively help relive pain, a patient may be referred for further treatment to these clinics. As well as a medical doctor and specialist nurses, the pain clinic team may include a clinical psychologist or counsellor. These professionals can help and give guidance on issues that affect mood and self-confidence.

Relaxation therapies

These therapies can help in the management of chronic back pain. By relaxing the mind and muscles, pain can be relieved. Meditation and deep-breathing exercises are examples of a relaxation therapy. Relaxation tapes can be found in most shops and can be used at home.

Acupuncture

Acupuncture has been used in Chinese medicine for thousands of years and there are various theories on how it works. A practitioner inserts thin needle just under the skin. Always use a qualified practitioner.

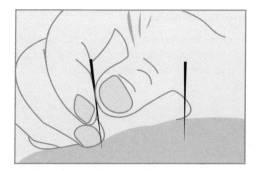

Fig. 6.3 Acupuncture.

Complimentary therapies

These are very much an individual choice but can be useful. Therapies such as aromatherapy and reflexology may help with relaxation and pain. Aromatherapy uses essential oils from plants, which are applied to the skin by massage or inhalation. It is important to ensure that the practitioner involved in giving advice on complimentary treatments is fully qualified and a registered member of that profession. Check with your GP or other health professional first.

Lifestyle changes

Lifestyle changes may have to be made so that pain can be managed. Some consideration should be given to actively taking steps to make daily lifestyle activities easier. Attitudes to pain and lifestyle are important. It is worthwhile to think about each and to work out how best to manage it. Planning ahead and deciding if an activity has to be done that causes pain means that painkillers can also be planned. The individual can ensure painkillers are taken beforehand and plan a period of rest after the activity. For example, when ironing, look at what causes the pain after this activity. It may make a difference if the ironing board is adjusted to the correct height, sitting instead of standing to iron, only doing a little at a time, and having frequent breaks. Adapting the situation to cause less pain can make a difference if the activity is planned. Pacing yourself and your activities makes it easier to cope with pain.

Pain-management techniques

It may happen that even with various treatments, pain is still there. Pain management involves knowing yourself and how your pain affects you, and developing ways of managing your life in order to lessen the impact and to stop the pain from worsening.

Summary

◆ Most osteoporotic fractures occur after a simple injury or fall, some of which could be prevented. Identifying patients quickly after such fractures is essential to pick up those at risk of future fractures. The development of fracture liaison services in the UK has been an extremely valuable way forward.

◆ Hip fractures are a major cause of morbidity and, sadly, mortality. The economic costs of these fractures are also high. Prevention of such fractures must be our main goal when managing those with osteoporosis.

7

The multidisciplinary team

> ➡ Key point
>
> All members of the multidisciplinary team aim to enable the person with osteoporosis to cope with the condition and to reduce the risk of fracture.

People with osteoporosis are likely to come into contact with different health-care professionals who can help address many of the problems encountered with the condition. This chapter gives a brief description of some members of the multidisciplinary team and their roles.

The general practitioner (GP)

The GP is usually the first point of contact for the patient and is central to providing care for the person with osteoporosis. The GP will refer a patient to a hospital specialist for diagnoses of osteoporosis. Osteoporosis may, however, be diagnosed following a fall or fracture when the patient attends a hospital for treatment and is referred to osteoporosis specialists. Once a diagnosis is reached, the GP will be guided by any treatment recommendations made by the specialist. The GP will refer the patient back to the hospital outpatient department, if there are any changes requiring specialist intervention.

Hospital specialist

Specialist doctors practice within a defined field of medicine and have vast experience and additional qualifications within that field. A hospital specialist will be able to diagnose osteoporosis, and recommend future care and drug therapy. The specialist may be a consultant or specialist doctor practising in a number of specialities, including rheumatology, endocrinology, gynaecology, or medicine for the elderly. The specialist will review the patient in the outpatient clinic and will discuss all aspects in reaching diagnosis of the condition. The patient will be asked questions about their medical history. The specialist will order tests considered relevant, such as blood tests and a bone density scan. Once a diagnosis is made, the specialist will write to the GP and make recommendations on treatment and care of the patient. The patient may be asked to attend the outpatient clinic regularly for review by the specialist. Orthopaedic surgeons are also hospital specialists and are often responsible for managing fractures when they occur but rarely advise on drug therapy for osteoporosis.

Osteoporosis specialist nurse

An osteoporosis specialist nurse is a registered nurse with additional experience and postgraduate training in the specialty. The osteoporosis specialist nurse can provide information and advice on all aspects of the condition, including lifestyle, treatments, control of pain due to fractures, and prevention of falls. Providing support to those who have osteoporosis is an integral part of the role of the specialist nurse. Some specialist nurses manage telephone advice lines and this is one of the ways that support can be provided.

The osteoporosis specialist nurse manages and organizes programmes of education for patients who are newly diagnosed with the condition. Some osteoporosis specialist nurses may also review patients in outpatient clinics. In addition, the osteoporosis specialist nurse provides education and advice for other health professionals, both within the hospital and in the community.

Physiotherapist

Physiotherapists are registered practitioners trained to help patients mobilize to their optimum levels by implementing exercise programmes to improve function and mobility. The specialist, GP, or osteoporosis specialist nurse may refer the patient for assessment by a physiotherapist to improve mobility or balance, or for exercise advice to build up weak muscles that are causing pain or discomfort.

Physiotherapy has an important role, both in helping control pain and in recovery following a fracture. By showing how to improve muscle tone and strength, balance, co-ordination, and posture improve, which in turn helps with pain and confidence to resume normal activities.

Occupational therapist (OT)

If the patient has difficulty managing activities related to their daily living, they may be asked if they would like to see an OT. The OT can visit the patient at home to assess if any home modifications can be made that will make difficult activities easier for the patient. Occupational therapists can also assess the home environment and give advice on how to make the home safer in order to avoid falls. The OT is extremely valuable in the prevention of falls in the elderly.

Pharmacist

A pharmacist is a healthcare professional trained in the prescribing of medications. Pharmacists have excellent knowledge on the methods of action of medications and their possible side-effects and interactions. Pharmacists can help greatly in explaining the rationale of treatments to sufferers with osteoporosis, in ensuring the optimal method of taking medications, and in highlighting to medical staff where concerns exist of problems with taking medications appropriately.

Summary

◆ A multidisciplinary team working together will give the best care for patients with osteoporosis.

◆ Many specialist groups have skills that greatly enhance the management and well-being of the patient diagnosed with osteoporosis.

◆ These health professionals work together and refer amongst themselves to provide optimal care.

8

Future developments in osteoporosis management

The last 15–20 years have been exciting times for osteoporosis management. As indicated elsewhere in this book, the techniques for diagnosing people at risk of osteoporosis have increased dramatically, and the quality of the risk assessment has been also markedly improved. New treatments have become available with good evidence that they reduce fractures, the important consequence for many who develop osteoporosis. As indicated elsewhere, hip fractures are the most expensive and devastating type of fracture, and methods to prevent these are particulary needed.

At present treatments for osteoporosis are targeted at those who have very low bone density and/or who have suffered a recent so-called fragility fracture. A fragility fracture is one that occurs when a patient falls from no higher than a standing position or suffers a fracture without injury at all. Treatment under these circumstances usually requires a measurement of bone density before it can be considered valuable or acceptable to treat. However, it is slowly becoming recognized that treatment of high-risk individuals can be undertaken safely and effectively without necessarily measuring bone density. In February 2008 the World Health Organisation issued a report entitled *WHO scientific group on the assessment of osteoporosis at primary health care level,* which identified the way forward for assessment of patients with osteoporosis, based on a combination of risk factors outlined elsewhere in this book, and bone density measured at the hip. This report is based on the examination of very large databases of both men and women from populations around the world. Based on the analysis of these populations, a risk factor scoring method was drawn up and then validated or examined in a further set of data from populations to confirm how correct the initial models were. The work has, therefore, been done very carefully. The publication describes how the work was carried out and the resultant output produces equations that allow the calculation of the fracture risk of both major osteoporotic fractures and hip fractures, separately, over the coming 10 years for men and women aged 40–90 years of age. Clinicians looking after patients at risk of osteoporosis can use an online questionnaire, which could be used also by the general public, as it is available on the world-wide web at http://www.shef.ac.uk\FRAX. On the website, at the moment, patients, but more often their doctors, from China, France, Italy, Japan, Spain, Sweden, Turkey, the United Kingdom, and the USA are able to calculate 10-year probability of major osteoporotic or hip fracture with or without measurement of bone density. When bone density is included in the calculation this will be a measurement at the hip, particularly the femoral neck.

The value of calculating these probabilities is because in many countries, perhaps including the United Kingdom, the risk of fracture will become the major deter-minant of whether or not it is appropriate and cost-effective to treat a man or a woman who has either suffered a fracture after the age of 40 or who has major risk factors for osteoporosis. Doctors may need to use the tool to assess whether a patient requires a bone density scan or whether they can be treated.

The risk factors that are assessed include a hip fracture in on the patient's parents, current smoking, and use of steroid tablets for inflammatory conditions, rheumatoid arthritis, and a variety of causes of secondary osteoporosis (outlined in Chapter 2), as well as those who take more than three units of alcohol per day. In the near future, country-specific tables using these probabilities will become available to clinicians and these will allow doctors to decide whether or not a patient might benefit from the measurement of bone density to help with the assessment of risk or whether indeed the risk is so high that they can progress directly to drug treatment to prevent fractures as outlined in Chapter 4.

In many countries in Europe, this approach will be sanctioned by the health authority for defining the people who can most usefully receive treatment to prevent osteoporosis, but it is not yet clear whether the National Institute for Health and Clinical Excellence (NICE) will sanction such an approach for use in the United Kingdom. The great advantage of the new method of assess-ing risk will be to target treatment at those at the highest risk thereby prevent-ing fractures in those who have most to gain, while providing such a facility at reasonable to cost to health budgets.

Summary

♦ Fracture risk-assessment tools are becoming available to help doctors and their patients assess their individual risk of future fracture. This will allow targeting of therapy to those who have the greatest risk of fracture.

Appendix—helpful organizations

British Society for Rheumatology
Bride House
18–20 Bride Lane
London
EC4Y 8EE
Tel: 020 7842 0900
http://www.rheumatology.org.uk

International Osteoporosis
Foundation (IOF)
9 Rue Juste-Olivuer
CH-1260 Nyon
Switzerland
Tel: 44229940100
http://www.iofbonehealth.org

National Osteoporosis Society
Manor Farm
Skinners Hill
Camerton
Bath
BA2 0PJ
Tel: 0845 450 0230
http://www.nos.org.uk

National Osteoporosis Foundation
1232 22nd St NW
Washington DC
20037-1202
Tel: 202 223-2226
http://www.nof.org

Osteoporosis Australia
Level 1
52 Parramatta Rd
Forest Lodge
NSW 2037
Sydney
Tel: 61 29518 8140
http://www.osteoporosis.org.au

Glossary

Algorithm	A procedure for solving a problem.
Analgesia	Medication or treatment for relief of pain.
Bisphosphonates	Medications that act by slowing down the action of osteoclasts, the bone cells that remove the old and worn out bone cells. Alendronic acid, risedronate, and ibandronate are examples of bisphosphonates.
BMD	Bone mineral density.
Bone density scan	See DXA.
Colles fracture	Fracture of wrist bones.
Dowagers hump	See kyphosis.
DXA	Dual energy X-ray absorptiometry (DXA) or bone density scan is a type of X-ray used to diagnose osteoporosis.
Fracture	Broken bone.
Genetic	Genes (biochemical code determining inherited characteristics).
Hormone	A chemical substance secreted in a gland and carried in the blood to have action on other body functions.
Kyphosis	When the shape of the spine is curved forwards, sometimes called Dowager's hump.
Metabolism	Chemical processes in a human body essential to maintain life.
Mortality	The state of being liable to die, the number or frequency of deaths.
Opioid	A drug that acts like opium.
Orthopaedic	Branch of medicine concerned with bones and joints; surgeons rather than physicians.

Osteopenia	A measure of bone mineral density that is lower than normal but not so low as to be in the range of osteoporosis.
Osteoblasts	Cells that build new bone.
Osteoclasts	Cells that remove the old, damaged, and worn out bone.
Osteomalacia	A disease characterized by painful softening of the bones, usually caused by lack of vitamin D.
Paget's disease	A chronic bone disease where overactivity of bone turnover leads to increase and irregular formation of bone.
Systemic	Pertaining to or affecting the body as a whole.
Vertebra	A bone in the spine.

Index

The index entries appear in word-by-word alphabetical order.
Page references in italics indicate figures and tables.